Collins *gem*

Cholesterol Counter

Kate Santon

First published in 2007 by Collins, an imprint of HarperCollins Publishers Ltd.
77-85 Fulham Palace Road
London
W6 8JB

www.collins.co.uk
Collins is a registered trademark of HarperCollins Publishers Ltd.

8 7 6 5 4 3 2 1
11 10 09 08 07

A catalogue record for this book is available from the British Library.

ISBN 978-0-00-725979-3

Collins uses papers that are natural, renewable and recyclable products made from wood grown in sustainable forests. The manufacturing processes conform to the environmental regulations of the country of origin.

Edited by Grapevine Publishing Services
Designed by Judith Ash
Printed and bound in Italy by Amadeus.

This is a general reference book and although care has been taken to ensure the information is as up-to-date and accurate as possible, it is no substitute for professional advice based on your personal circumstances. Consult your doctor before making any major changes to your diet.

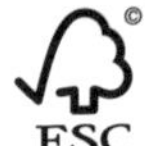

Mixed Sources
Product group from well-managed forests and other controlled sources
www.fsc.org Cert no. SW-COC-1806
© 1996 Forest Stewardship Council

FSC is a non-profit international organisation established to promote the responsible management of the world's forests. Products carrying the FSC label are independently certified to assure consumers that they come from forests that are managed to meet the social, economic and ecological needs of present and future generations.

Find out more about HarperCollins and the environment at
www.harpercollins.co.uk/green

CONTENTS

INTRODUCTION

Cholesterol has a terrible reputation. However, despite the fact that increasing numbers of people are being advised that their cholesterol levels are too high and that they should try to reduce them, there's a lot of confusion about what this means and how it should be achieved.

It has been estimated that as many as 70 per cent of people over the age of 45 in the Western world have levels of blood cholesterol that are too high to be considered healthy – levels that put them at risk. A significant number of younger people are thought to be developing high levels, or to already have them. High levels of cholesterol in the blood are important because they substantially increase the risk of developing cardiovascular disease (CVD), a term which includes coronary heart disease (CHD) and stroke. A high cholesterol level *alone* is likely to be responsible for 46 per cent of all premature deaths from coronary heart disease in Britain.

Doctors often hand out basic diet sheets when patients have high blood cholesterol levels and may provide some initial information – and, in some cases, drugs – though this is often relatively rudimentary. There are some widely publicised products available, from spreads and breakfast cereals to prescription drugs, which can be used to lower cholesterol levels with varying degrees of effectiveness. As a result it is recognised that having a high cholesterol level is potentially dangerous, but exactly what this means and how it affects us is less well understood.

Most of us have heard of 'good' and 'bad' cholesterol, though just what that means is even less frequently discussed. It is easy to be left with the impression that you just have to eat the right foods, containing the right kind of cholesterol, while avoiding others (eggs are often quoted). Ideas like these are widespread but they are completely incorrect: you can't eat 'good' cholesterol and you don't have to avoid eggs.

There is so much 'information' out there that the soundness of the basic advice that doctors give can be drowned out by extraneous noise. Making basic changes to your diet and lifestyle can help reduce your cholesterol levels, and those changes are not complicated.

Another fact that is often obscured is that cholesterol is actually necessary; we all need it in order for our bodies to function. The risk associated with it comes into play when levels are too high, and the aim of managing your cholesterol levels is to reduce that risk, thus lowering your chance of developing cardiovascular disease and having a heart attack or stroke.

WHAT IS CHOLESTEROL?

Fat is transported around the blood as lipids – a collective term for all fatty substances in the blood. Lipids include phospholipids, trigylcerides (which you will probably first encounter in a blood cholesterol test), waxes and sterols. Cholesterol is a sterol, doubtless the best known. It's a waxy substance in the blood, mostly manufactured and/or processed in the liver, and none of us can live without it. In small amounts it is essential for our health, and it is found in every single cell of the body.

Cholesterol builds and maintains the membranes of cells as well as the insulating sheaths that run around nerve fibres, sending messages to and from the brain and around the body. It occurs in very high concentrations in these cells, which protect the nervous system and brain, and is therefore especially important when those systems are developing. It's one of the base ingredients of hormones such as oestrogen and testosterone; of cortisol, which helps us adapt to stress; of aldosterone, which ensures that the body regulates salt and potassium levels; and of Vitamin D, without which the body cannot absorb and use the calcium needed to build and maintain healthy bones.

Cholesterol is used in the liver to make bile acids, which are then stored in the gall bladder. They enable the body to dissolve fats from food and thus help the digestive process to work more effectively. This action also ensures that the vital fat-soluble vitamins (A, D, E and K) can be absorbed as well. So, while having too much cholesterol can be very bad, life without it would be impossible.

Moving cholesterol around the body

In order for cholesterol to get to where it is needed, it has to be moved from the liver and transported around the body in the bloodstream. Rather like oil and water, fats and blood plasma don't mix, and cholesterol doesn't dissolve in blood either. To make it possible for fats to move in the circulatory system, they are packaged into particles covered with proteins. The proteins do more than just protect the fat, though; they seem to act rather like email addresses, sending the particles in the right direction. These particles, known as lipoproteins, are able to flow along with the blood, mixing easily with it. The lipoproteins contain some cholesterol, which helps to stabilise them, and by this means cholesterol is carried around the body too. Lipoproteins can be compared to car transporters, couriers or delivery trucks, dropping off some items and picking up others.

Lipoproteins vary and are classified – generally – according to the balance of fat and protein they contain. Those with more protein and less fat are denser and heavier than those which have more fat than protein, which have been described as light and fluffy. As far as cholesterol goes, the most important lipoproteins are high-density lipoprotein (HDL), the more fat-laden low-density lipoprotein (LDL) and the very low-density lipoprotein (VLDL). The first two – HDL and LDL – have become known, somewhat inaccurately, as 'good cholesterol' and 'bad cholesterol' respectively. Those shorthand terms have arisen because of how these lipoproteins behave and the effects they can have.

Cholesterol and dietary fats are moved from the digestive tract to the liver by another lipoprotein, chylomicron, which is made in the small intestine. But most of the body's cholesterol is manufactured in the liver, and this is also where it is packaged for transport together with triglycerides. Briefly, the liver collects fatty acid fragments from the blood and makes new fatty acids and cholesterol from them. It also seems to monitor the amount of dietary cholesterol taken in; if your diet includes a lot, your liver may make less, and vice versa.

Triglyceride-transporting VLDL particles are made in the liver. They carry excess fatty acids from the liver to the adipose tissue – the body's fat stores – passing through capillary walls into the surrounding tissue where the free fatty acids are released for storage. After these free fatty acids are released, LDL particles are formed from what remains.

LDL or 'bad cholesterol'

Low-density lipoproteins are the main carriers of cholesterol. They contain a higher proportion than other lipoproteins and move about 70 per cent of the cholesterol in circulation to the body tissue where it is needed. They vary in size and number, and have a protein on the surface which matches a receptor site on the surface of a cell, like a key matching a specific lock. This allows the LDL to pass into the cell where it dissolves and releases the cholesterol it contains.

Most of the cholesterol needed by our cells – for instance, to make cell membranes or manufacture sterol compounds such as hormones – is supplied in this way. In the genetic disorder called familial hypercholesterolaemia (see page 15), LDL particles are restricted from entering the cells.

If LDL levels are high, however, not all of them are removed from the blood in this way, and some of them end up in the wrong places. They can pass through artery walls, where they are collected by scavenger cells known as macrophages (which also take up other excess particles, like micro-organisms). This is the start of the process that leads to the development of 'atherosclerotic plaques' – fatty deposits that narrow the arteries and can eventually block them, leading to heart attacks and angina.

LDLs also vary in stability and, to follow the delivery truck comparison, some are more likely than others to drop off their cholesterol parcels in this way.

High levels of LDLs in the blood are strongly associated with an increased risk of heart and circulatory disease – and this is the reason why LDLs have become known as 'bad cholesterol'. The lower your LDL levels, the better for your health. In fact, even if your overall cholesterol levels are low, you may be at risk if your LDL levels are high.

HDL or 'good cholesterol'

High-density lipoprotein particles, the smallest lipoproteins, are made in the liver and intestines from the remains of LDLs. They collect excess cholesterol from the cells and carry it back to the liver for processing, in a system known as reverse cholesterol transport. It also appears that HDL is able to stop cholesterol building up in newly formed deposits on artery walls.

HDL might also have some kind of antioxidant properties (see page 51). Unstable, oxidised LDL is particularly likely to damage artery linings and spark off a series of reactions which eventually lead to the development of clots which block the blood vessels. Some scientists have suggested that antioxidant activity can stop the oxidation process beginning in the LDL particles, and that this may be the most important way in which HDL works.

Whatever the precise mechanics, having a high level of HDL in the blood is clearly associated with having a lower chance of developing cardiovascular disease, and this is why it has become known as 'good cholesterol'. The higher your HDL levels are, the better for your health. Women tend to have slightly higher levels than men, at least until the menopause.

What happens next?

The excess cholesterol which is returned to the liver can either be recycled into more lipoprotein particles or converted into bile acids. These then move into the gall bladder, from where they pass out of the body in the stools – so not only does the liver manufacture cholesterol, but it also removes the excess. Reducing the recycling option appears to be part of the way in which soluble fibre reduces cholesterol (see pages 48–50). It is also the mechanism by which stanol and sterol esters work (see pages 56–7).

Where does cholesterol come from?

Only a very small amount of cholesterol comes directly from your diet; most – about a gram a day – is produced in your liver from the food you eat. Small amounts are also made in almost all the body's cells but the liver can actually provide all the cholesterol needed by the body.

However, if your diet is high in saturated fats it can cause your liver to produce more of the LDL particles, those which have become known as 'bad cholesterol'. The effect that diet has on blood cholesterol does vary from person to person and seems to be genetically determined but, broadly speaking, a diet high in saturated fat increases the amount of cholesterol circulating in the blood, while one that is higher in unsaturated fat reduces it.

Some foods contain cholesterol, but not all – another misconception. It is found in food that has an animal origin, or that is derived from animal sources: meat and poultry, fish and shellfish, dairy products and eggs. There is no cholesterol in egg white, though, nor in any plants or products derived entirely from plants: none in sugar, none in avocados, none in potatoes, none in raspberries, none in nuts or seeds… Some of these foods are, however, high in saturated fat. For example, coconuts and their derivatives – like coconut milk and oil – are very high in saturates.

Unless you already have a serious heart condition, have been specifically advised to do so by your doctor, or have certain blood disorders, you are unlikely to have to monitor closely the amount of purely dietary cholesterol you take in. Watching the quantity and type of fat you consume is much more important.

CHOLESTEROL TESTS

Mass screening for cholesterol levels is usually thought unnecessary. Blood cholesterol is usually only measured when there is some compelling reason to do the test. Having a high cholesterol level in itself does not cause symptoms – though sometimes some signs can be observed. These could include yellow cholesterol deposits in the skin around the eye, known as xanthelasmas; tendon xanthomas, which are swellings on muscle tendons, particularly noticeable on the Achilles' tendon at the back of the heel; and a corneal arcus – a white ring in the outer part of the cornea. This last sign has little significance in older people but should be regarded with suspicion if it is present in someone in their thirties and forties; it can be picked up during a routine eye examination. If you think you have any of these signs, it is worth discussing it with your doctor.

FAMILIAL HYPERCHOLESTEROLAEMIA

Sometimes, an abnormally high blood cholesterol level can be caused by an inherited condition called familial hypercholesterolaemia. This often remains undiagnosed but it is thought that about 120,000 (or 1 in 500) people are affected in Britain. People with this genetic disorder may suffer from heart attacks and strokes in their thirties and forties, and anyone with a family history of early deaths from CVD should have a cholesterol test. Sufferers from this disease have a 50:50 chance of passing it on to their children.

If you have any form of CVD already, your doctor should be testing and monitoring your cholesterol levels. Otherwise you should ask your GP to refer you for a test if you have any of the following:

- A family background of early coronary disease.
- A family history of familial hypercholesterolaemia.
- Any other CVD risk factors, such as diabetes or high blood pressure, being overweight or obese or smoking, especially if you are over 35.

Blood tests are taken to determine cholesterol levels. To give a complete picture (known as a full lipid profile), this should be a fasting blood test – one where you don't eat or drink anything other than water for 12 to 16 hours beforehand. By this time any food you have eaten will have been completely digested and have no effect on the result. A non-fasting test only measures total cholesterol and HDL.

The test is best done professionally – at your GP's surgery, in hospital or as part of a general medical check-up. There are portable machines, desk-top analysers, which work with blood from a simple finger prick, but more often a full blood sample will be taken. It is possible to buy simple home kits or have finger-prick tests done in some pharmacies, but some of the home kits are not particularly accurate.

What the test results show

The blood is analysed to establish how much cholesterol is present in a litre of blood – that is, how much cholesterol is being carried by the lipoproteins at the time of the test – and the figure is shown in millimoles per litre, or mmol/L. This is how the figures will appear if you get a printout of your test from your doctor – such as a total cholesterol figure, for example, of 5 mmol/L. If you are told that your cholesterol is '5', then this means 5 millimoles per litre. This is an internationally recognised standard unit, used everywhere except in the US. There, cholesterol is measured in milligrams per 100ml (or decilitre), abbreviated to mg/dL, and the equivalent to 5 mmol/L would be 195mg/dL.

Sometimes an initial test is done to establish a total cholesterol level and a more detailed breakdown is only undertaken if necessary, when the total figure – which includes a combination of LDL and HDL – is above a certain value. More often, though, you will have a full lipid profile done. That will include figures for both LDL and HDL, as well as for triglycerides and a total cholesterol to HDL ratio.

There are official guideline figures available, though there is some debate about whether or not they are too generous, at least for people with other conditions like diabetes. At present it is recommended that the total cholesterol level should not exceed 5 mmol/L, nor should LDL levels be greater than 3 mmol/L. Some prominent societies and charities concerned with cardiovascular disease believe that it would be better if these figures were each lowered by one, to 4 mmol/L and 2 mmol/L respectively.

As a basic generalisation:
• A cholesterol level higher than 6.5 mmol/L is a high risk factor for heart disease. It's been estimated that about 20 per cent of the UK population have levels of 6.5 or above.
• A figure lower than that yet greater than 5 is a moderate risk, and below 5 is low risk. The average figure in the UK is 5.2 mmol/L, and in the Western world as a whole it is higher, at 5.9.
• If you have a level above 7.8 mmol/L your risk factor is three times greater than someone with a level of 6.5.

There are a number of other factors – such as whether or not you smoke – that are taken into consideration when assessing risk (see page 24).

Some people have a high level of total cholesterol because they have a high level of 'good' HDL – over

2 mmol/L – so the ratio between total cholesterol and HDL is also taken into consideration to look at the overall balance. This is often considered to be the most important figure derived from a cholesterol test.

To take one example, someone with a total cholesterol level of 5.2 and an HDL reading of 1.43 would have a total cholesterol/HDL ratio of 3.63.

Total cholesterol ÷ HDL = TC:HDL

If your total cholesterol was a high 7.5 and your HDL 1.1, your TC:HDL would be 6.81. That would not be good news: a total cholesterol to HDL ratio of more than 4.5 is associated with increased risk. The lower your ratio, the higher the overall levels of HDL in your blood and the better for you.

Triglycerides

Triglycerides are likely to be mentioned when you have a cholesterol test. Almost all of the fats in the diet are triglycerides – three fatty acids bound together by glycerol – and they provide us with energy. Triglyceride is transported to the cells by VLDL particles and most is stored, but some is also found in the blood. Just like cholesterol, triglycerides are necessary; and just like cholesterol, too much triglyceride can be bad for your circulatory system. It is associated with pancreatitis, an inflammation of the pancreas which is both serious and painful.

The precise role of triglycerides in the development of coronary heart disease is often debated, as the results of clinical studies have been inconsistent, but it is likely that a raised level of triglycerides, more than 2 mmol/L – combined with a high level of LDL and a low level of HDL – can increase the risk of developing coronary heart disease. People with diabetes are particularly vulnerable, as are those who are overweight or who drink too much alcohol.

Finally, the link between high triglyceride levels and developing CHD seems to be stronger in women. The key to controlling blood triglycerides is comparatively straightforward – eat healthily, include oily fish or fish oil in your diet, keep slim and keep fit.

Test variability

Certain factors can affect cholesterol readings and levels can also fluctuate naturally, varying from one day to the next. For this reason any suspiciously unusual, unexpected or high readings will probably lead to a re-test, and you may be tested several times before any drugs are prescribed.

THE PERFECT SCORE

As a basic summary, here are the blood lipid levels you should aim for:

- A total cholesterol of 5 mmol/L or less; preferably 4.
- LDL levels of 3 mmol/L or less, preferably 2.
- HDL levels above 1, preferably above 1.5 (women's levels are naturally higher).
- Triglycerides of 1.5 or less.
- A TC/HDL ratio of well below 4.5.

There is some variation between sample-testing labs, but this is small and international measures are under way to ensure that all laboratories are comparable. In addition, desk-top anaylsers show more variations than do full blood samples.

Other factors can affect your precise cholesterol levels. Some are determined by who you are, while others are more general.

- **Age and sex**. In men, average blood cholesterol rises until the age of about 50, when it begins to fall a little. Once women reach the menopause their levels go up.
- **Menstrual cycle and pregnancy**. Levels can vary by as much as 9 per cent over the menstrual cycle, with

the highest ones occurring in the first half. They also rise in pregnancy, and both increases are a result of hormonal changes.

- **The way the test is taken.** Leaving a tourniquet on for a longer time – if it is difficult to find a vein, for instance – can lead to an apparently higher figure.
- **Time of year**. There are some seasonal variations, but figures can be about 3 per cent higher in winter. It is not known exactly why this is.
- **Illness, surgery and major trauma**. Levels fall dramatically in these circumstances, and stress is thought to be the reason why this happens. Even a simple viral infection can lead to a reduction of up to 15 per cent.
- **Cancer**. With any form of cancer there is usually a fall in blood cholesterol levels.
- **Drugs**. Some medicines can affect the levels of blood lipids, especially triglycerides. This is another reason to get a test done by someone who has access to information about your medical history.

The causes of high cholesterol

Some medical conditions – like familial hyper-cholesterolaemia, some kidney and liver diseases, diabetes which is not well controlled, or having an underactive thyroid – can cause high blood cholesterol levels, as may some unrelated medicines.

You can't do anything about your family history, age and sex. However, for most people the main causes are related to diet and lifestyle, and you can change these.

Your cholesterol levels may be high if you:

- Eat a diet high in saturated fat – and, for some people, possibly one also high in cholesterol.
- Don't take much exercise, which appears to increase LDL levels.
- Are overweight or obese, which seems to increase LDL and decrease HDL levels.
- Drink excess alcohol.

It is important that you address these risk factors if you have high blood cholesterol levels, because the risk attached to not doing so is substantial.

HIGH CHOLESTEROL: THE RISKS

Cardiovascular disease (CVD) is common and often fatal: it causes a higher proportion of deaths below the age of 75 than any other disease. In the UK, it is the main cause of premature death in men – that is, dying before you are 65. Coronary heart disease (CHD) causes about 26 per cent of male deaths below the age of 75, and almost 20 per cent of deaths in women under that age; another 14 per cent or so die from related conditions.

CVD is also one of the major causes of poor health; the British Heart Foundation estimates that over 2.7 million people in Britain have either had a heart attack or suffer from angina. The UK's death rate from heart disease is one of the highest in the world, though it is falling slightly, and the same is true of the US. However, rates are going up in some developing countries, and worldwide CVD remains the most common cause of death, with around 10 million deaths a year attributable to it.

Generally, where the average cholesterol level is low – in some parts of the Far East, for instance, it is only 3 mmol/L as opposed to the West's average of 5.9 mmol/L – the rate of cardiovascular disease is also low.

Cholesterol levels aren't, of course, the only risk factor for developing CVD, but they are significant. Here are some of the others:

- Smoking.
- Not doing any physical activity (or very, very little).
- Being overweight, especially if the excess is principally around your middle.
- Drinking a lot.
- Having high blood pressure or diabetes.
- Having high levels of the amino acid homocysteine,

which seems to damage artery walls when present in high quantities (this may be why some people with low cholesterol have heart disease).

- Being older.
- Being male.
- Having a family history of heart disease.

Calculating your risk of developing cardiovascular disease can be quite technical; there are CVD and CHD risk calculators, but talking to your doctor is the best place to start. Though there has been some recent controversy about methods of determining risk, the fact remains that the more risk factors you have, the greater your chances of developing CVD.

Some of these general risk factors you can't change, but some you can. Of those, the most significant appears to be your cholesterol level, so it does make sense to try and do something about it. The staggering fact is that high cholesterol alone may be responsible for nearly 50 per cent of all premature deaths due to heart disease in the UK.

Cholesterol and CVD

The term cardiovascular disease – meaning disease relating to the heart or blood vessels – covers a whole range of circumstances in which undue strain is put on your arteries or other blood vessels, or on the heart itself. The heart is the pump at the centre of the bloodstream and has to work efficiently in order for us to survive. The body has a number of mechanisms to try and ensure that the circulatory system is kept in a state of good repair and less susceptible to damage – but they are not foolproof.

Blood travels to the heart through the coronary arteries and these become narrower with age. This comes about largely because of the effects of a normal 'Western' lifestyle – a diet high in fats and lack of everyday exercise. Blood vessels can also become blocked when too much cholesterol in the blood causes a fatty deposit known as an atheroma, or a cholesterol plaque, to be laid down within the artery walls. It then hardens and a scar is formed, a condition called atherosclerosis or coronary artery disease, often referred to as your arteries 'furring up'.

An atheroma gets bigger over time, which can result in thrombosis (the formation of a blood clot) and a reduction in blood flow through the vessel. Large clots can block arteries completely or break up unexpectedly, both of which have devastating and catastrophic consequences and apparently come with no warning – sudden heart attacks, when they prevent blood from reaching the heart, or stroke, when they stop it reaching the brain.

There are also some chronic conditions associated with hardening arteries which can have a serious impact on your overall quality of life. The most well known are:

- **Angina**, a type of chest pain that comes on with exercise – or, indeed, with simple exertion – and diminishes with rest. Angina is often an early sign of more serious heart disease. The pain is usually felt across the chest, but can occur in the shoulders and arms, even the jaw and throat; it generally lasts for less than 10 minutes. It can be brought on by excitement, stress or by suddenly eating a large meal (the rate of angina attacks and heart attacks rises over the Christmas period), as well as by exercise. It should always be investigated by a doctor. The situation can deteriorate, with attacks becoming more frequent and occurring even when the sufferer is at rest. The pain of a heart attack has been described as 'crushing and severe'; it lasts longer than angina pain and cannot be relieved by resting.
- **Peripheral vascular disease**, obstruction of arteries in the legs, which can lead to severely restricted mobility. The first signs may be an aching in the leg muscles when walking, that is relieved by rest, but

symptoms can worsen until the pain is severe and continuous.

• **Transient ischaemic attacks**, or TIAs. These are sometimes called mini-strokes and are caused by a temporary interruption in the blood supply to the brain due to a small clot. They generally don't last for long – about 24 hours – and are marked by slight brain dysfunction; they should always be taken seriously, as they are a sign that there is, potentially, a more major stroke in the offing. In fact, they are so reliable as an indicator of trouble ahead that the UK's Stroke Association has recently launched an awareness campaign, and any suspicion of a TIA should lead to an immediate medical check.

If your blood cholesterol – and particularly your LDL level – is high you are more likely to develop these conditions. As causes of premature death, they can largely be prevented. The link between them and blood cholesterol is very clear, so now is the time to try and do something about it.

MANAGING HIGH CHOLESTEROL

There are clear benefits to reducing high cholesterol. Up until about 30 years ago this was not so evident, but study after study since then has confirmed it. Lowering your blood cholesterol can have substantial effects, especially if you are at high risk of developing cardiovascular disease, and particularly coronary heart disease. It slows the development of arterial disease and improves survival rates.

There are essentially two ways of approaching the task of lowering your cholesterol levels, and which one your doctor recommends will depend on your personal situation. The first and most common one is just to modify your lifestyle: change your diet and increase the amount of exercise you take. The second is drug treatment combined with lifestyle modification. By remembering that the aim is to reduce your risk of death or developing a disabling illness, not just a desire to get your cholesterol down to some theoretical limit, you will have a powerful motivating factor working in your favour.

Lifestyle changes

Here is a basic summary of the lifestyle recommendations:

- Eat a healthy and varied diet (see pages 33–57).
- Reach and maintain a healthy body weight (see pages 58–61).
- Stay active or take up exercise (see pages 61–3).
- If you smoke, you are greatly increasing your risk of CVD and you should try and stop – but you doubtless know this already.

Prescription drugs

When you get the results of your cholesterol test, your doctor may talk to you about prescription drugs, that can reduce the levels of blood cholesterol. Whether or not you need to take them will depend on your overall risk of developing CVD and not just on your cholesterol level. People who have high blood cholesterol but who are otherwise fit, who are not overweight and who don't smoke or drink excessively will probably not be offered these drugs. If you already have diabetes or cardiovascular disease as well as high cholesterol, you are highly likely to be given them – and you should take them.

The most common group of drugs which lower blood cholesterol levels are statins, and the ones most frequently prescribed are simvastatin (Zocor) and atorvastatin (Lipitor). They reduce the amount of cholesterol produced in the cells of the body, making it necessary for them to obtain it from that which is circulating in the bloodstream. More LDL particles are taken up by the cells, removing more of the 'bad' LDLs from the blood, and thus – logically – reducing overall blood cholesterol levels.

Statins are less effective at increasing the amount of 'good' HDL or at reducing triglycerides, but they may help to improve the condition of artery walls. If you are prescribed statins, you will normally be told to take them in the evening, as there is a slight overnight increase in the amount of cholesterol manufactured. Your treatment should be monitored and your cholesterol measured regularly to check how you are doing, and your prescription may be altered accordingly.

It is now possible to buy lower doses of simvastatin in pharmacies without a prescription. You should not even think about doing this if you already have diabetes, familial hypercholesterolaemia, CHD or any other CVD risk factors. In these circumstances you must seek your doctor's advice as you will probably need a higher dose than is available over the counter, and you should be under medical supervision anyway.

You should also not take statins if you are pregnant or breast-feeding. Basically, don't take them if you don't need to. It is worth noting that recent work done at the University of Toronto has shown that a diet high in the right foods – one rich in fruit and vegetables, lean meat, tofu, barley and particularly almonds, oats and oily fish – can be as successful as statins at reducing cholesterol levels.

Some people may experience a few minor side effects with statins, among which are indigestion, muscle pain and disturbed sleep, but they are usually fairly trouble-free drugs. They are, however, among those which can react with grapefruit. This is not a myth; grapefruit can boost the blood levels of quite a lot of drugs, increasing their effect and also increasing the chance of experiencing unpleasant side effects. It is essential that you avoid grapefruit and grapefruit juice if you are taking statins.

There are some other prescription drugs used to treat high blood cholesterol, but they are generally less effective or have more frequent side effects. They include ezetimibe, a cholesterol-absorption inhibitor (and relatively recent addition), fibrates (which have a better effect on triglycerides than statins and also increase the amount of HDL in circulation) and nicotinic acids (not often used in the UK, largely because of the side effects). Other new treatments are in development.

Finally, none of these is an alternative to a healthy diet and sensible lifestyle. If you are eating foods high in saturates and taking no exercise, you still need to change this to reduce your risk of CVD even if you are taking medication such as a statin. Eating healthily will enhance the effect of the drugs, so you should make every effort to do so.

EATING FOR THE GOOD OF YOUR HEART

Making dietary changes is one of the most important things you can do to reduce your risk of CVD, by both reducing your cholesterol levels and your weight. It should also have an impact on another risk factor, high blood pressure, and may help you to reduce others, such as sedentary lifestyle. If you feel better in yourself, exercising is much more fun and you're more likely to want to do something energetic. But making serious changes to habitual ways of eating, to the food you have come to love even though it may be bad for you, is often difficult. Is it really necessary?

There is very substantial evidence that it is. Two huge scientific studies – the Seven Countries Study and the Lyons Diet Heart Study – have borne this out unequivocally. The first of these was led by Dr Ancel Keys, a highly respected American physiologist, in the 1960s. Initially intrigued by reports of differing rates of CVD between the US and southern Italy, Keys began investigating. The most significant and immediately obvious distinction was in the general diet of the two populations, and it was clear that the only sector of southern Italian society whose incidence of CVD approached that of people in the US were the upper classes – the people whose diet most closely resembled that of the Americans. Deaths from CVD among other social groups were much lower.

Keys, a real pioneer, then began more detailed work in Naples, including assessing cholesterol levels – and discovered that the level of blood cholesterol was lower in most of his Italian subjects than in the US. His work in Italy prompted research in several other countries with widely differing death rates from CVD, and so the Seven Countries Study began. That showed clearly, among other things, that the percentage of calories in the diet from saturated fat was linked to the development of – and deaths from – heart disease.

The US and Finland, which had the highest rates of death, also had the highest average consumption of saturated fat. The Mediterranean island of Crete had the lowest rate of death from heart disease, as well as the longest overall life expectancy. The diet of the Cretans was what is now known as a typical 'Mediterranean diet', with lots of vegetables, fruit, unrefined-grain carbohydrates and olive oil, and with much smaller quantities of meat and full-fat dairy produce. They also ate more fish, particularly oily fish.

The Lyons Diet Heart Study is more recent; it began in 1988 and was undertaken to see if the Mediterranean diet could reduce the incidence of further heart attacks among a large number of people who had already survived their first one. Half of the people in the study were asked to follow the diet which the American Heart Association was recommending, while the other half followed a clearly defined Mediterranean diet.

The study had only been running for two and a half years when the supervising ethics committee ordered it to be stopped early as the beneficial results of the Mediterranean diet were so definite: a 70 per cent reduction in deaths, and that was in deaths from all causes. Several years later the researchers checked up on the study's participants again and discovered that the benefits were still in evidence (there was even a reduced risk of cancer). Many of those who had been on the Mediterranean diet for the research project liked it so much that they were still following it. Since then other studies, such as the huge Nurses' Health Study in the US, have confirmed individual findings from both of these research projects.

The Mediterranean diet has many advantages in terms of the health of your heart, and of the health of the rest of your circulatory system. It also has several other good points which make it easy to adopt. It incorporates a huge range of delicious foods, so it is simple to follow and does not become boring over time. There is a wide variety of cooking styles and traditions to pick up on: much of the cooking around the Mediterranean follows the same principles, from Morocco to the Middle East and from Southern France and Italy to Greece and Egypt, so there is plenty to inspire you to change. At the same time, the general principles can easily be adapted to other cultural traditions, such as the cooking of the Indian subcontinent. And the closer you can get your own diet to the basic model, the better for you.

There are some basic principles which you can adopt.
• Reduce fat, or foods that are particularly high in fat, and use unsaturated oil, preferably olive or rapeseed oil rather than the saturated fat alternatives.
• Eat less red meat and more fish, especially oily fish.
• Fruit and vegetables are the centre of the Mediterranean diet, so increase the amounts of those and eat at least five portions a day, if not more.
• Refined-grain products (white bread and flour, white rice) are eaten comparatively rarely; wholegrains are

much more common, and the overall diet is high in fibre.

• Full-fat dairy products should be eaten much less frequently than is usual in the average Western diet.

• Alcohol is drunk in moderate quantities, often with food.

• For the good of your heart you should also watch your salt intake, using less salt both in cooking and at the table. If you cut the amount of ready meals and processed food you eat you will automatically reduce the quantity of salt you consume, as many of these foods have high levels.

• The classic Mediterranean diet also tends to be lower in sugar. Yes, there are sweet puddings and honey is popular throughout the region – but sugar is used nowhere near as frequently as it is in the UK.

Understanding fats

If you have high blood cholesterol levels your doctor will probably give you some unequivocal advice on the fat in your diet. Eating a lot of food high in saturated fat will increase the amount of cholesterol circulating in your blood, thus increasing your risk of CVD. On the other hand, if your diet is high in unsaturated fats it will reduce the amount of cholesterol circulating and lower your level of risk. Changing the type of fat you eat is one of the most important and vital alterations you can make to your diet, and it has a much greater impact on blood cholesterol levels than lowering the amount of dietary cholesterol (cholesterol included in the food you eat). For most people, monitoring fats is more important than monitoring cholesterol.

This is because different types of fat have different effects on your blood cholesterol. Saturated fats seem to encourage your liver to produce more LDL particles, while blood cholesterol levels are lowered when mono-unsaturated fats, in particular, are used instead. Most foods have a combination of fats, with one or another being dominant. Olive oil, for instance, is usually described as a monounsaturated fat because that is the most prominent type of fat which it contains, at 73g per 100g, but it also contains polyunsaturates (8.2g) and saturates (14.3g).

Here's a guide to fat types, together with some information about them and the effects they have.

Saturated fats raise both LDL and HDL levels, and intake should be reduced. Saturated fats are solid at room temperature. Some types of saturates seem to be worse than others, with those from dairy products boosting LDL levels the most. Then come those in beef fat, poultry skin, and finally those in cocoa butter

> **SOURCES OF SATURATED FATS**
>
> They are particularly found in: whole milk; cream; butter; lard; suet; hard cheeses; full-fat ice cream; red meat; sausages; poultry skin; meat pies; a lot of processed foods; pastry; coconut milk, oil and coconuts themselves (the saturated fat in coconut is a different type to that found in foods of animal origin; at present the exact role of this kind of saturated fat is being debated, so it is worth being cautious). Palm oil is also high in saturates, so watch for it in ingredients lists – check out oatcakes and peanut butter, for instance. Biscuits and cakes are often high in saturates, and so are some powdered cappuccino drinks. A lot of snack foods are high in them too, though at present many manufacturers are changing to other kinds of fat.

and chocolate. This is not, unfortunately, a licence to eat huge quantities of chocolate!

Polyunsaturated fats fall into two categories – omega-3 and omega-6 fatty acids, which are sometimes (especially in the US) called *n*-3 and *n*-6 fatty acids. They may lower both LDL and HDL levels. A normal diet usually includes enough omega-6, but omega-3 levels can generally do with a boost. Omega-3 fish oils may also affect the 'stickiness' of the blood making it less viscous and therefore less likely to form clots, thus reducing the risk of stroke and heart attacks. There is also an indication that they might offer some protection against abnormal heart rhythms.

GOOD SOURCES OF OMEGA-3 ARE:

- Fish oils; rapeseed oil; olive oil; spreads made using these oils; linseeds (also known as flaxseeds); soya beans; nuts; eggs.

GOOD SOURCES OF OMEGA-6 ARE:

- Soya and sunflower spreads; corn oil; safflower oil; sunflower oil; soya oil.

These vital fatty acids are liquid at room temperature. They are not made by the body and must be derived from food; because of this they are known as essential fatty acids. There is enough omega-6 in a normal healthy diet without the selection of appropriate foods but in the past – beginning in the 1980s – spreads with a high level of omega-6 were considered particularly healthy as an alternative to saturated fats like butter. This is no longer the case; they have now been shown to increase inflammation in the body when compared to monounsaturated fats, such as olive oil, so opt for spreads high in those instead. However, most people need to increase the quantity of the omega-3 they consume by making deliberate choices and, preferably, eating one portion of oily fish a week. Some foods are supplemented with omega-3s: you may find additional omega-3 in cereals, orange juice, special milk or margarines. You can buy eggs from chickens fed a diet high in seeds; these are much higher in omega-3 than ordinary eggs and are sold as such; there is also some evidence that organic eggs have higher levels. It is recommended that omega-3 from both fish and plant sources should be included in the diet, so that means nuts and oils as well as oily fish. Some foods, like eggs and fortified spreads, contain both types.

If you take a fish oil supplement to make sure you get enough omega-3 you should check that the dose it provides is adequate. Look for the EPA (eicosopentanoic acid) and DHA (docosohexanoic acid) figures – to gain the benefits, you need 450mg of combined EPA and DHA every day. Most gel capsules provide much less; a 1000mg capsule of fish oil, for instance, might contain 180mg of EPA and 120mg of DHA. A teaspoonful of cod liver oil, though it may seem initially off-putting, provides more than double that, so do check the labels on supplements and make sure you know what you are buying.

NB: Fish liver oils are high in vitamin A and should be avoided during pregnancy except under specific medical advice.

Monounsaturated fats are thought to lower LDL levels and raise HDLs, and are recommended over polyunsaturates for this reason. These are the fats you should generally choose, whenever possible, instead of saturated ones. Like polyunsaturates, they are liquid at room temperature. They also seem to enhance the good, anti-inflammatory effects of omega-3 fish oils.

Rapeseed oil is often sold as vegetable oil in the UK so check labels (it may also be called 'canola oil'). This has a neutral taste which some people may prefer to olive oil, and such a bland flavour may also be more appropriate when cooking certain dishes.

SOURCES OF MONOUNSATURATED FATS

They are found in: olive oil; rapeseed oil; groundnut or peanut oil; spreads made from these oils. They are also present in peanuts; almonds, cashews, walnuts and most other nuts, as well as in peanut butter (but watch out for added palm oil) and avocados.

Trans fats are the one other type of fat that needs to be considered when you are deciding whether your diet is healthy or unhealthy. Like saturated fats, trans fats can raise the levels of LDLs and a high intake of them can significantly increase the risk of developing CVD.

It is often thought that trans fats are entirely artificial but some do occur naturally; they are present in very small quantities in meat and dairy products. Most of the trans fats encountered are, however, artificial creations produced during hydrogenation, a process used to convert liquid vegetable fats into semi-solid substances. These are extremely useful to the food industry and are found in products ranging from margarines and spreads to biscuits and cakes. Producers and manufacturers are cutting back on trans fats due to the now well-known overall risk to public health – some studies have suggested they are even worse for you than saturates – but you are still likely to come across them in smaller amounts.

Anything described as a 'hydrogenated fat' or a 'partly hydrogenated fat' in a list of ingredients is a trans fat, and should be avoided wherever possible. Read the labels, and be aware. Avoiding pre-packaged and processed foods altogether is the safest option.

Dietary cholesterol probably need not be restricted if you are eating a good, balanced diet. You might be advised, however, to eat foods containing it in moderation, perhaps no more than three or four times a week (though be prepared for this advice to change, as continuing research is currently stressing the lack of impact dietary cholesterol actually has on blood cholesterol). You will find detailed information in the listings section of this book, but there are some broad guidelines opposite.

Choosing fats

Remember that the most important thing you can do to reduce your blood cholesterol is to cut down on the saturated fat in your diet. The main reason why foods that are high in dietary cholesterol seem to have little effect on overall blood cholesterol levels is because they are also low in saturated fat.

You can reduce the amount of saturated fat you eat relatively painlessly by reducing the quantity of full-fat dairy products and red meat in your diet, and by removing any chicken or turkey skin. Cutting out fast foods, junk foods, many ready meals and processed foods will also help enormously by taking away a lot of unnecessary saturates and trans fats from your diet. You will never eliminate saturates completely,

SOURCES OF DIETARY CHOLESTEROL

- **No-cholesterol foods (and those with trace amounts):** plants or purely plant-based foods have none at all. Vegetables and vegetable oils are cholesterol-free, as are fruits, nuts, grains, egg-free pasta, rice, egg white and sugar. Small traces are found in some breads and breakfast cereals, and foods made with butter – like croissants – have higher levels. Some crisps have a trace.
- **Low-cholesterol foods**: tinned fish in vegetable or olive oil, white fish (so long as it has no coating); very lean meat and skinless poultry; low-fat dairy products. Most oily fish is relatively low, too.
- **Medium- to high-cholesterol foods:** full-fat dairy products including butter, cheese and ice cream, many ready meals, processed foods and manufactured goods such as cakes and anything with pastry; meat and fish products including deli meats and smoked mackerel; the fat on meat and poultry.
- **High-cholesterol foods**: offal, including liver and foods that contain it like pâtés and some deli goods; egg yolks and foods containing them like mayonnaise and chocolate mousse; shellfish, particularly squid, prawns and scampi; fish roe.

nor should you attempt to do so; don't forget that good sources of mono- and polyunsaturated fats like olive oil contain some saturated fat. But you should try and change the emphasis of your diet to one which is better for your health, and improve its overall balance.

One other thing: we all need fat in our diets, despite the fact that some weight-loss diets demonise it. It provides energy and insulation and helps us to feel full after meals, but it also has less obvious functions. Some vitamins are only fat-soluble; fat is part of every cell membrane and forms part of the protective myelin sheath around the nerves, allowing them to transmit information (brain tissue is rich in fat, too). It's an internal shock absorber, protecting our organs if we fall or hurt ourselves in the same way that the more visible fat padding protects the bones. And it's a constituent of hormones. All of these are reasons why nobody should take things to extremes when it comes to lowering fat intake.

Very low-fat diets are inadvisable, particularly for people who are at risk of developing CHD or who already have it, so don't try and cut it out. It is very difficult to tolerate extremely low-fat diets for any length of time.

Facts and figures

At present it is recommended that no more than 33 per cent of daily food intake should be in the form of fat, with no more than 10 per cent coming from saturates. One gram of fat contains 9 calories, so if you eat a total of 2000 calories a day, that would be 73 grams of fat. Assuming that you eat the government's recommended levels of calories (most of us probably eat more), men should have up to 95g of fat a day, including no more than 30g of saturated fat; women up to 70g, with no more than 20g of that being saturates. To calculate how much your current diet contains, you would need to keep an accurate food diary, weighing and measuring everything, then work out the exact fat content of what you had eaten. You probably have a fairly good idea of whether it is high in fat without going to such lengths, but be realistic.

Read nutritional information panels on packaging and use them as a guide. If a label says something has 20g of fat per 100g, or has more than 5g of saturates, then it's got a lot of fat in it and should be avoided. When it says 'low fat' on labels it means that the product should contain less than 3g of fat per 100g – but check the other ingredients, as sometimes these low-fat products are high in sugar or salt to compensate for the reduced taste.

Fibre

Dietary fibre comes from plant-based foods such as grains, pulses, vegetables and fruit, and there are two kinds – soluble and insoluble. There is no fibre in meat, poultry, fish or in dairy products and eggs; nor is there any in sugar. Dietary fibre is made of carbohydrates that cannot be digested. It has a definite link with lower rates of CVD, and especially CHD.

Insoluble fibre absorbs water and keeps you feeling satisfied after food. It also helps food to move through the digestive system and can prevent digestive disorders from developing. It is found in the outer layer of vegetables and the husks of whole grains.

Soluble fibre is found in foods like oats and barley, pulses, fruits and vegetables (the pectin in fruit, for example). It has been shown to lower cholesterol levels significantly by reducing the amount of cholesterol absorbed from the intestine, binding dietary cholesterol and some of the bile salts so that they cannot be reabsorbed by the liver and recycled. Study after study has confirmed that people who have lots of soluble fibre in their diets have a much lower chance of developing heart disease. It can also make you feel fuller after a meal, just like insoluble fibre. Another benefit of soluble fibre is that it helps reduce the body's absorption of glucose, keeping blood sugar levels steadier than low-fibre foods do.

As far as reducing cholesterol is concerned, oats are the focus at the moment. They contain beta-glucan, which is seemingly better at lowering cholesterol than other soluble fibres, but there is still much work to be done in establishing just why this is so. Going by some advertising campaigns, you might almost think that oats were magical in the effect they have on cholesterol. They are very good for you, but only as part of a healthy diet.

People who eat a lot of wholegrain products – wholemeal bread, brown rice, wholewheat cereals, for example – have been shown to have much lower rates of CVD. This may be partly because they are consuming more fibre, but wholegrain cereals have other benefits too. Among other things they contain many more trace elements than their refined equivalents, as well as antioxidant minerals and vitamins, like vitamin E.

Nutrition experts recommend that adults consume 18g of fibre a day.

Fruit and vegetables

Eating more fruit and vegetables is the mainstay of all cardio-protective diets and is not just associated with benefiting your heart and circulatory system; lower rates of cancer are found when fruit and vegetable consumption is high. Studies have also shown that eating more fruit and vegetables can lower blood pressure as well – another significant CVD risk factor – and the effect is particularly marked when they are combined with a diet that's low in saturated fat.

Vegetables and fruit are so important for good health that the World Health Organisation has recommended a daily consumption guideline of at least 400g, roughly equivalent to the 'five a day' highlighted by recent health campaigns.

Fruit and vegetables are important because of the many useful substances they contain. They are often high in fibre, comparatively low in calories (unless cooked in a way that increases calories massively, like deep frying), rich in antioxidants, in essential vitamins and minerals, and full of phytochemicals.

Some of these are particularly useful for CVD prevention. The B group vitamins: folic acid, a vitamin present in leafy vegetables, pulses and oranges, works with vitamins B6 and B12 to reduce blood levels of homocysteine. High levels of this amino acid appear to damage artery walls, increasing the risk of stroke and heart attacks.

Antioxidants

Antioxidants have been getting a lot of attention recently but, as with cholesterol, there is some general confusion about them. Certain vitamins, minerals and phytochemicals (chemicals from plants) have an ability to stop oxidation, a chemical reaction which can lead to damage and deterioration of the cells. The main antioxidants are vitamins A, C, E and beta-carotene (a form of vitamin A) and the minerals selenium and zinc. Flavonoids from fruit, particularly citrus fruit, are also vital, as are specific phytochemicals such as lycopene (found in tomatoes, watermelon and red grapefruit) and quercetin (present in apples, the onion family and black or green tea). There are others.

The role of antioxidants and their specific relation to the prevention of heart disease is being studied at present, and recent work has shown that rates of CHD are worst in countries where people have low antioxidant levels. Fruit and vegetables, so strongly emphasised in the Mediterranean diet, are a major source of antioxidants; so are wholegrains. While more research is still needed on exactly why it works, the protective effect of eating lots of fresh fruit and vegetables cannot be doubted.

There has been some interesting research about the effects of antioxidants on blood lipids. LDLs can change chemically by oxidation, which increases their uptake by macrophages, the scavenger cells in arterial walls. These are the beginnings of atherosclerotic plaques, those fatty deposits that can eventually lead to blocked arteries. It looks as though antioxidants can prevent this process from happening – at least in the lab – and there have been some suggestions that the beneficial effects of HDL may be a result of its antioxidant properties. This is, however, a developing field.

The best way to improve your intake of antioxidants is to eat more fruit and vegetables. Supplements are available but tests have shown them to be ineffective; they may perform in the test tube, but the body is a different matter. Buy some fruit instead.

Chocolate

Chocolate contains antioxidant polyphenols, which are responsible for stopping dairy fat going rancid.

They are why chocolate can be kept well without going off, and have been known about for many years. Now the flavonoids in chocolate are thought to have benefits in terms of the antioxidant impact they have on LDLs, as well as other benefits derived from their ability to relax artery linings and affect immune function positively. They also have anti-inflammatory properties.

These flavonoids come from the cocoa beans but, in practice, not a lot of cocoa bean is present in much of the chocolate available on the high street. Milk chocolate, for instance, doesn't contain many cocoa solids. Select plain chocolate with over 70 per cent cocoa when you fancy a bit of chocolate – but bear in mind the calorie load. The picture is, however, even more complicated. The flavonoid content of chocolate is variable and changes with the type of bean used, the particular plantation it was grown on, how it was prepared, the growing conditions and even, apparently, the weather at the time of harvest.

Alcohol

It is thought that alcohol, particularly red wine, has beneficial effects because of its antioxidant content. You don't have to drink wine if you don't want to just because it featured in the original Mediterranean diet

– and you should drink it in moderation anyway – but there may be some advantages. Drinking a small amount of alcohol daily does appear to protect you from CVD, and it is thought that it actually reduces mortality from heart disease.

In France, heart disease has historically been at surprisingly low levels, given that the overall diet is quite rich in saturates and that many people have other risk factors like smoking. This is known as the 'French paradox', and the role of wine drunk with meals has been suggested as a possible explanation. Reservatol, found in the skin of the grapes that make the wine, was often described as being responsible, but it is now thought that its levels are probably too low. It may be the alcohol in the wine, rather than phytochemicals, which is effective, in which case any alcohol would have similar effects. The quantity of procyanidins in red wine do, however, improve the dilation of the blood vessels.

Alcohol can reduce the stickiness of the blood, improve insulin response and minimise damage to the arteries from inflammation. It reduces LDLs and increases HDLs, but its benefits only outweigh its disadvantages if consumption is in moderate amounts (see pages 82–3).

Coffee

Some people are concerned about coffee, as there have been reports that it can raise cholesterol levels. In practice this is only relevant when you drink a lot; and men who drank ten or more cups a day were indeed found to have higher blood cholesterol levels than those who drank fewer. The effect on cholesterol seems to depend on how the coffee is prepared, with Turkish coffee and cafetière coffee evoking more of a response than filter or instant coffee. Moderate intake is not associated with any risk to your health and there may be some benefits in terms of the effect caffeine seems to have on kidney stones and gallstones, so don't worry about it unduly.

Soya

Eating soya protein every day has been shown to reduce LDL cholesterol significantly – but the effect does not seem to be the same for everyone, and the levels that are required to bring about a beneficial response are quite high – 25g per day. Lower amounts do not have the same effect, and eating or drinking 25g would be difficult for many people; half a litre of soya milk, for example, provides only 20g.

In addition, almost 33 per cent of the UK population are unable to convert the phytochemicals in soya into a form that affects LDL. Soya's benefits are not just confined to the cardiovascular system, as soya beans are an excellent source of the plant form of omega-3. Experimenting with soya products like tofu and soya yoghurt will certainly do you no harm, and tofu can be a great substitute for meat in a stir-fry or soup. While soya is certainly interesting, it is probably not worth making radical changes to include it in your diet.

Sterol- and stanol-enhanced foods

There are many products available in supermarkets which have added ingredients that are supposed to help lower your cholesterol. There are two factors that should be considered:

- Firstly, they only work if they are part of a healthy diet and lifestyle. They are not a substitute for it. If you normally eat fairly unhealthily and just use these, making no other attempt to change what you eat, they will not work.
- Secondly, they are designed for people with high cholesterol. The official advice is that only people who have high blood cholesterol levels should eat these products on a regular basis. People with normal cholesterol should not do so; this is particularly important for children and women who are pregnant or breastfeeding.

The official recommendation is that you can help to lower your high blood cholesterol levels by changing your diet without adding these 'functional foods', and that if you do eat them, you should check the labelling carefully to ensure that you don't use too much.

When products are advertised as 'helping to lower your cholesterol' or being 'specifically developed to soak up cholesterol', keep your eyes open and read the small print. That will usually say something like '…as part of a diet low in saturated fat and a healthy lifestyle' – and this is the critical part. It's the lifestyle changes that make the difference. Remember that these products may *help*, but they are not magic wands. It is our responsibility, as individuals, to change our diet and lifestyle for the better.

TACKLING OTHER RISK FACTORS

Though high levels of blood cholesterol are a major risk factor for developing cardiovascular disease, they are not the only one. Nor are they isolated from some of the others, such as being overweight or obese, or taking very little exercise. Improving the amount of exercise you take, for example, can have a direct impact on your cholesterol levels as well as on your overall fitness.

A healthy body weight

Body weight and high blood cholesterol don't always go hand in hand but they are frequently linked, and if you are overweight you should be addressing the issue. There are many reasons why being overweight is bad for your heart and circulatory system. Among others, if you are overweight you are more likely to develop type 2 diabetes and high blood pressure, both of which, separately and jointly, make you more liable to develop artery-blocking atherosclerotic plaques.

We tend to think of body fat as inactive – 'it's just flab' – but it isn't. It generates substances known as adipokines, which can increase inflammation of the arteries and also speed up the development of atherosclerosis. This can constitute an independent risk, quite apart from whether or not someone also has high blood cholesterol. The good news is that you don't have to lose all of your surplus weight to affect adipokine production.

Your doctor may use the BMI or Body Mass Index to assess how overweight you are. Working out your BMI is comparatively simple, involving the use of a calculator, weighing scales and a tape measure. You need to know your weight in kilograms and your height in metres (no shoes!) in order to determine your BMI. Divide your weight by the square of your height to get your score.

An example makes the process clearer. If you are 1.65m tall and weigh 80kg, it looks like this:
1.65 x 1.65 = 2.72
80 ÷ 2.72 = 29.4
This last figure is your BMI.

BMI is assessed on a scale. If your BMI is less than 18.5, you are underweight. You're at a healthy weight if it is between 18.5 and 24.9, overweight if it's between 25 and 29.9, and obese if it's above 30 (there are gradations of obesity above this, too).

There are problems with the BMI, though – among other things, it doesn't take into account muscle, which weighs more than fat, or overall build – and that's why doctors also like to look at waist measurements and the waist-to-hip ratio when assessing cardiovascular risk.

Excess fat that is stored around the waist can increase the chance of developing CVD. It is associated with higher levels of inflammation of the arteries as well as increased insulin resistance, and this leads to an added tendency to develop type 2 diabetes and high blood pressure as well as increased triglyceride and cholesterol (but lowered HDL) levels. Waist measurements are often used by themselves.

- If you are female and your waist is over 80cm you're at some risk, and at more if it's over 88cm; you should aim for less than 80cm
- If you are male and your waist is over 94cm you're at some risk, and at more if it's over 102cm; you should aim for less than 94cm.

The measurements should be taken straight round the middle: over the navel and not above or below any bulge, of course.

Another way of assessing cardiovascular risk from weight is to look at the waist-to-hip ratio. You've got your waist measurement; now measure around the widest part of your hips, also in centimetres. Divide your waist measurement by that of your hips.
For example:
78 ÷ 107 = 0.73
This gives you your ratio. You are looking for a value of 0.83 or below if you're a woman, and 0.90 or below if you're a man. If your waist-to-hip ratio is higher than those figures, then your size can be considered as another risk factor.

Changing a previously unhealthy diet to one that is healthier will probably bring about a gradual decrease in weight. Deliberately 'dieting', especially using fad or crash diets, is to be discouraged in any circumstances. Some diets will put additional strain on your cardiovascular system. If you need to lose weight, bear in mind the basic rule that energy in is related to energy out. If you put more energy into your body as food than it uses to keep itself going and in physical activity, then you will put weight on. Take in less energy (and/or use more), and you will lose weight.

See how it goes while also making the dietary changes needed to reduce your blood cholesterol. Don't try to reduce your weight too quickly if there's no improvement, but just cut the amount you eat by about 500 calories a day at first, and take more exercise. If there's still no gradual reduction, start calorie counting. Keep to between about 1400 and 1600 calories per day if you're female and roughly 1600–1800 if you're a man, rather than trying anything more extreme.

Physical activity

Inactivity is dangerous; it's a major risk factor for stroke and almost doubles the risk of having a heart attack. And there's evidence that being sedentary (sitting watching TV, for instance) increases food intake, usually food that's high in fat, salt or sugar – just the sort you want to avoid.

Basically, people who take some exercise are less likely to develop heart disease, but you don't have to get to an Olympic level. The greatest advantages come from moderate exercise; pushing your physical activity to extremes does not cause a corresponding increase in the benefits gained. The exact reasons why exercise works are not entirely obvious – but the fact that it does is clear. Just one exercise session can raise HDLs by about 10 per cent, and reduce triglycerides by an average of double that figure.

Anyone who has done very little exercise for some time should seek their doctor's opinion before starting. This is particularly true if you have a pre-existing heart or blood-pressure problem; in those circumstances, you should always consult your GP about the programme you plan to undertake. This is also true if there have been any premature deaths from CVD in your family or if you are very overweight or obese. Make sure you exercise under some sort of supervision, at least at first. If you decide to go to a gym, then be completely frank with the staff there about any medical conditions and take their advice about what you should do, and to what intensity you should do it.

Don't push yourself too far. The good news is that you don't have to take out gym membership. All you have to do is make sure you get 30 minutes of exercise a day, and even things like dancing count, as do brisk walking or gardening, so long as whatever it is leaves you slightly breathless. If you are not used to taking any exercise at all, then build up slowly. If you feel any pain when you exercise, stop immediately and consult a doctor.

High blood pressure and salt

Blood pressure makes it possible for the necessary supply of blood to reach every cell in the body, so we all have it and need it. As with cholesterol, though, problems arise if it is high. High blood pressure is also known as hypertension.

When you have your blood pressure taken you will get a reading which looks something like 120/80 (that's a good blood pressure, by the way). The larger figure is the systolic pressure, the increase in pressure you get with every beat of the heart. The smaller figure is the background blood pressure, called the diastolic pressure. Blood pressure is variable, both during the day and according to circumstances, but if your blood pressure is regularly over 140/90 you will be told that you have high blood pressure. You should take this seriously, as it is a major risk factor for CVD.

There are several things you can do to lower your blood pressure. One of the first – again – is making sure that you eat healthily. The Mediterranean diet, recommended for the effects it has on levels of blood cholesterol, can have a significant impact on hypertension when you also reduce your salt intake. Losing weight can be of benefit, as can increasing physical activity. So can stopping smoking and reducing excessive alcohol consumption. In some cases you may be prescribed medication.

Blood pressure tests that give a high reading should always be repeated because of natural variability – there is, for example, a syndrome known as 'white coat hypertension', which means a patient's blood pressure has risen due to the stress of seeing a doctor.

In some specific circumstances, such as if you have diabetes, your doctor may give you different blood pressure targets than the ones listed opposite.

BLOOD PRESSURE

There has been some debate about exactly where the boundaries of ideal, normal and 'high normal' blood pressure should be drawn, but here's a broad guide.

- If your systolic blood pressure is between 130 and 139, and your diastolic reading is between 85 and 89, your blood pressure is classed as 'high normal'.
- If your systolic blood pressure is less than 130 but more than 120, and your diastolic reading is between 80 and 85, your blood pressure is normal.
- Your blood pressure is at optimal levels if your systolic blood pressure is less than 120, and your diastolic reading is less than 80.
- If your blood pressure is over the 'high normal' level, you have hypertension.

Some people's blood pressure is particularly sensitive to salt. The average intake in the UK is 9.5g a day, and the official recommendation is that this should be reduced to 6g a day or less. You may wish to go further, as some important trials have shown that cutting back is highly beneficial. We need about a gram a day and excess is excreted, but not before the surplus salt has pulled water from the body's cells.

So where does the salt in our diets come from?

- 15 per cent occurs naturally in unprocessed food.
- 15 per cent is added during cooking or at the table.
- And the rest – an astonishing 70 per cent – comes from manufactured or processed foods such as ready meals, tinned food, breakfast cereals, biscuits…

To reduce your salt intake, reduce the amount of processed foods you eat, and always rinse the salt off foods tinned in brine, such as tuna or olives.

Smoking and heavy drinking

All smokers know they are putting their health at risk, but they may not be clear exactly how it can affect their circulation. Nicotine constricts arteries, reducing the blood supply not just to the heart but to other tissues as well. Carbon monoxide from any smoke inhaled reduces the amount of oxygen the blood can carry, and the combination of lower oxygen delivery and reduced blood supply can lead to serious cell damage. Nicotine and free radicals from inhaled smoke can damage the artery walls, thus increasing the development of atherosclerosis.

Smoking also raises blood pressure and lowers HDL levels, to such an extent that improving diet and lifestyle while still smoking will completely negate the changes you have made. It really does make sense to stop, even though it can be very difficult. There is plenty of help out there. Read *Collins Gem Stop Smoking*, or consult your GP.

While drinking some alcohol may help your cholesterol levels, consuming excessive amounts will increase your risk of developing CVD. It can cause excessively high blood triglyceride levels, as liver cells stop the normal processing of fats while they deal with the alcohol (which has been described as a 'powerful cell poison'). Overall cholesterol levels can rise as a result. Alcohol causes raised blood pressure as well, but makes someone who drinks excessively resistant to the drugs used to treat hypertension. And these are just the CVD-related problems from excess alcohol consumption: there are many, many more.

Stress

Everyone knows that stress is bad for your blood pressure, but sustained high stress levels can also have other effects. In fact, they can increase your risk of developing CVD by more than double. The stress hormones adrenalin and cortisol can damage blood vessels and encourage atherosclerosis, and raise the levels of fibrinogen, a protein which encourages blood clotting. It can be difficult to address excessive stress – or even, sometimes, to recognise it in yourself – but it is always worthwhile.

Homocysteine

High levels of homocysteine have been clearly associated with CHD, though they are much less widely known about than other risk factors. Homocysteine is a substance that is produced naturally by the body – it's a by-product of protein digestion – but high levels are dangerous. It has been recognised since the late 1960s, when the deaths of two small children from massive strokes provoked investigations. Both had genetic disorders which affected how their bodies processed homocysteine, and both of them had arteries which were clogged up with cholesterol. The link was initially dismissed, but having high levels of homocysteine is now widely recognised as a significant risk factor for developing heart disease or having a stroke.

Ensuring there are adequate amounts of the B vitamin folic acid, vitamin B6 and vitamin B12 in the diet is the key to controlling homocysteine levels, and the US Food and Drug Administration has been fortifying grain products like breakfast cereal with folic acid since 1998. Fortified products, particularly breakfast cereal, are now more widely available but fruit and vegetables also provide a good supply; so do certain other foods like yeast extract. Improving your diet should also enable you to control your homocysteine levels.

Vegans may need to supplement their diet with vitamin B12 tablets, as this is found naturally only in animal products, though some soya milks are also fortified with it.

FOOD SOURCES OF B VITAMINS FOR CONTROLLING HOMOCYSTEINE LEVELS

Here's a brief summary of the non-artificially fortified sources of these vital vitamins.

- **Folate:** beans and pulses; leafy green vegetables including broccoli; asparagus; sweetcorn; soya flour; liver (chicken liver is particularly high); yeast and yeast extract; oranges and various other fruits; wholegrains.
- **Vitamin B6:** offal; chicken and turkey; fish; pork; lamb; lentils; wholegrains including brown rice; potatoes; sweet potatoes; bananas; beans including soya beans; nuts and seeds; dark green vegetables.
- **Vitamin B12:** meat and meat products; poultry; fish and shellfish; eggs; milk and dairy products; yeast extract and fermented products like miso and shoyu (a small amount).

ADOPTING A HEART-FRIENDLY DIET

In practice, most people find it more convenient to follow general guidelines than chase after precise fat counts or detailed 'eat-this-next-Thursday' plans. Here are some basic rules to follow which reinforce specific elements of the Mediterranean diet and which will enable you to change your diet in the most painless way possible.

THE BASIC RULES

- Use monounsaturated fat, like olive or rapeseed oil, rather than butter or lard or even a polyunsaturated oil.
- Reduce the fatty foods in your diet and always choose lean meat. Remove poultry skin and cut back on red meat; increase the quantity of fish, especially oily fish – try to eat two portions a week.
- Watch dairy foods, cutting back full-fat ones either by eating less or exchanging them for lower-fat versions; change to skimmed milk.
- Eat at least five portions of fruit and vegetables a day, more if possible.
- Eat high-fibre foods such as wholegrains, pulses and beans rather than any lower-fibre equivalents.
- Drink alcohol moderately.

To avoid temptation, try to eat regularly and ensure that you don't allow yourself to get so hungry that your judgement lapses. If you plan your meals this is much less likely; planning makes it easier to ensure that you are sticking to the basic principles and eating for the good of your health. Take time to have a proper breakfast, plan what you are going to have for lunch and make a healthy packed lunch if you wish, and think about what you are going to have in the evening – you may want to take something out of the freezer before you leave the house, for example. Make sure that you have predominantly healthy food in your store cupboards, fridge and freezer and you will be on the right track.

Getting fat right

The first habits to break, and the most important ones, are those connected to fat. While it would be impossible and unnecessary to cut fat completely, you should make sure that you are taking in as little saturated fat as possible, and changing to monounsaturates wherever you can. So:

- For cooking, choose a monounsaturated oil, such as olive oil or rapeseed oil, and use less; an oil and water spray is very useful.
- Replace butter with a healthy spread (see pages 188–91 for advice on what to look for).

- Substitute chicken or fish for red meat a lot of the time.
- When you do eat red meat, trim off the fat.
- Always take the skin off poultry.
- Eat at least two portions of fish a week, at least one of which should be oily fish.
- Use semi-skimmed or preferably skimmed milk.
- Switch to low-fat dairy products or cut the quantity you use by half.
- Try microwaving, steaming, boiling, grilling or poaching instead of frying.
- If you roast meat, do it on a rack so the fat drains away, and don't roast potatoes or vegetables in the tray under the meat.
- Avoid high-fat snacks, such as crisps, cakes or sweets.
- Avoid processed food and ready meals as much as you can; this applies to vegetarians as well.

THE ADVANTAGES OF OLIVE OIL

Most oils are extracted using solvents whereas olives are compacted in presses to produce the oil without the use of solvents. The colour and flavour of olive oil bear witness to the antioxidant polyphenols it contains. Use a good olive oil as a salad dressing, or in circumstances where you will really taste the flavour, but buy a less special one for cooking.

Meat and poultry

In almost all countries that border the Mediterranean, meat is part of the meal rather than its main focus. Red meat and fatty meat products like sausages and bacon should be eaten in moderation, and they should always be cooked in a healthy way – grilled, for instance, rather than fried. Get into the habit of removing visible fat before cooking to reduce the likelihood of succumbing to temptation afterwards. Stir-frying is a great way to cook meat; you need lean meat to start with, and a little goes a long way once it is cut into the necessary small pieces. The leanest cuts of red meat are topside of beef, rump and fillet steak; pork fillet and loin steaks; and cuts of game, such as venison.

The dark meat of chicken is higher in fat than the white meat, but there's no reason to avoid it if you remove the skin. Again, cook poultry in the healthiest possible way to minimise saturated fat content: don't fry it in lots of fat and don't let it sit in a roasting dish but cook it on a rack instead.

Fish

Eating more oily fish is one of the principles of the Mediterranean diet, but exactly which fish should you go for? Broadly speaking, fish with darker flesh are oily fish. Mackerel, herrings, fresh tuna, trout, salmon, sardines and swordfish are all good choices, as are their smoked or (in some cases) tinned versions. Don't fry fish in lots of fat, though, or add a coating of batter or breadcrumbs; grill or bake it instead.

Some people object to the smell of fish cooking, but this can be largely avoided by either cooking it in the microwave or baking it wrapped in a foil parcel. And some fish, of course, doesn't have to be cooked: try flaking some smoked mackerel over a salad or having smoked salmon with wholewheat toast. All fish and shellfish contain some omega-3 fatty acids, but oily fish contain the most.

If you've already had a heart attack, it is highly recommended that you eat 2–3 servings of oily fish a week, or that you take an appropriate fish oil supplement. Concern has been expressed over the levels of heavy metals found in some fish, but the official advice is that the benefits still generally outweigh the risks.

Dairy products

Full-fat dairy products are high in saturated fat, so you should try to reduce this element of your diet. There are two basic options, and they are not mutually exclusive: either eat much less or substitute low-fat versions. When it comes to milk itself, it is best to adapt to skimmed milk. Changing gradually may be easier than a straight swap, giving you time to become used to the much less fatty taste, so try adapting to semi-skimmed first. There are some very good low-fat yoghurts available, though some of the flavoured ones may contain a lot of sugar, so check the ingredients.

Some reduced-fat cheeses are low in flavour or have a strange aftertaste, so you may prefer to keep buying full-fat versions and just using less. Some varieties of cheese are much lower in saturates than others, such as Feta, fresh Mozzarella and Camembert.

Don't eliminate dairy products completely; they are a valuable source of calcium and your health may suffer without it. Vegetarians who avoid dairy products should supplement their diets or use fortified products like soya milk with added calcium.

Eat more fruit and vegetables

This is a crucial part of any heart-friendly diet, indeed of any healthy diet. If you're not used to eating lots of fruit and vegetables, you don't have to jump straight to five portions a day. Build up to it, keeping five – or even more – as your aim. Eating one portion rather than none, or three portions rather than two, will still bring some benefits. Don't be tempted to stop at one, though, and don't rely on any vegetables found in ready meals or processed foods – but you can count frozen, dried or tinned fruits and vegetables as well as fresh ones.

The other thing to avoid is counting several portions of the same thing as separate portions – five apples in one day does not, strictly speaking, equal five portions. The aim is to get some variety. Note that potatoes do not count as a portion at all... here are some examples of what does.

- 150 ml fruit juice (a tumblerful)
- A bowl of salad leaves
- An apple, banana or pear
- A handful of cherries, grapes or berry fruit such as strawberries
- Two tablespoons of raw, cooked, tinned or frozen vegetables
- A large slice of pineapple or melon
- Two small fruits, like apricots, plums or satsumas
- A tablespoon of dried fruit or three dried apricots.

Just as five apples wouldn't do the trick, so you can't have a repeat portion of fruit juice or dried fruit and count it again. Fruit and vegetables are full of minerals, vitamins and antioxidants and that is why you need the variety – to ensure you get the maximum benefits. In the UK, the Stroke Association has been promoting an easy way to remember that fact, under the slogan 'eat a rainbow'. Basically, the wider the range of colours in the fruit and vegetables you eat, the wider the range of nutrients.

There are several easy ways of increasing your intake. Not only are salads good for you, but adding a bowl of salad to every meal is also a great way of taking the edge off your appetite. Salads can be as varied as you like, from simple green salads and sliced tomato salads to main course dishes which could involve tuna or cold chicken, grains and cooked pulses as well as a variety of salad leaves.

For really fresh salad, try growing your own baby leaves – the seeds germinate quickly in summer and you can keep cutting them over several weeks if you choose appropriate varieties. Some supermarkets sell 'living salads' in pots. Growing and using rocket will add a spicy, peppery taste. Be careful about dressings, though – a simple olive oil and vinegar or lemon dressing is the best option, but drizzle on the oil lightly rather than glugging.

Soup is a great addition to a heart-friendly diet – preferably home-made, as some commercial varieties are high in salt and sugars. When you make soup you retain the nutritional benefits of the ingredients, and soups which are either made with pulses or left whole and unblended will give you the maximum level of fibre.

You can easily increase your fruit intake by substituting fruit for less healthy snacks. Many fruits already come conveniently packaged in their own skin. Where the skin is edible – such as with apples and pears – you should eat it because of the additional fibre it contains, but always wash the fruit well first.

Fresh or dried fruit, can be added to breakfast cereals or salads, and makes a delicious starter to a main meal. Don't forget that fruit juice can count as one of the five portions, but do read labels and opt for the one with the lowest number of additional ingredients. Or buy a juicer and prepare your own fresh juices.

Increase fibre

Fibre plays an important role in reducing cholesterol, and the traditional Mediterranean diet is high in it.

Unfortunately most Western diets are not, and this is another area where change can have significant benefits. As you increase the amount of fruit and vegetables you eat, you will naturally increase the amount of fibre, both soluble and insoluble. However, it is still worth making extra changes, reducing the amount of refined-grain products you eat, adding wholegrains instead and incorporating more pulses into your diet.

When grains and flour are refined, many essential nutrients are stripped away, along with the fibre they contain. It is worth substituting wholemeal bread for white bread, brown rice for white rice, and a wholegrain breakfast cereal for a more processed one. Wholemeal pasta is another product worth considering. Cous-cous and bulghur wheat are frequently used around the Mediterranean, and these can also form a useful addition to your diet. They are not so high in fibre but, like other carbohydrates, they help to make your meal more filling.

The glycaemic index (GI) can be a useful guide to the fibre content of carbohydrates; those which are highest in fibre have a low or medium GI. This is an indication of the gentle effect they have on your blood sugar levels, itself a function of how quickly they are digested, and foods which are higher in fibre are digested more slowly. GI diets have received much publicity of late but they are not just another fad; they are a way of eating healthily. Following some of their suggestions – eating more fruit and vegetables, more slow-release carbs (the highest in fibre) and opting for monounsaturated fats – can also help to lower cholesterol. Keeping your blood sugar levels steady will help to improve your overall blood lipid profile.

Before you automatically increase the amount of fibre you eat, think about what your present diet is like. If it is light in fibre you should increase it gradually, or you may find that you suffer from digestive problems as your system adapts. Make sure you drink enough water as well. Don't immediately swap to very high-fibre food; change gradually. As a general rule, eat the skins of things like baked potatoes and cut refined white grain products from your shopping list.

One of the easiest ways to incorporate more fibre in your diet is to begin by adding it at breakfast. Switch to a high-fibre breakfast cereal, maybe trying out some of the latest ones based on oats or just opting for porridge. Do be careful about what you put on your cereal, though; skimmed milk should be used instead of fuller-fat varieties (once again, cut down gradually if you find it hard to swap straight over). Smothering wholemeal toast in butter would not be advisable either.

Pulses – beans and lentils – are often associated with stodgy vegetarian dishes. This is entirely the wrong impression and if you avoid them you are really missing out. They are great sources of both kinds of fibre – soluble and insoluble – and are also high in nutrients such as the B vitamins, including folic acid; vitamin E; zinc; calcium and iron. Pulses are low in fat, high in protein and are particularly useful when used to supplement a dish containing meat or fish.

The variety is enormous, from delicate *lentilles du Puy* to meaty chickpeas, and there is something for

COOKING BEANS

Dried beans should be soaked overnight before use; drain them and throw out the soaking water, cooking them in fresh, to minimise the chance of indigestion. Some varieties – kidney beans and their immediate relatives – need brisk boiling for 10 minutes before slower cooking but they are all straightforward to prepare.

everyone. In addition to dried beans, there are many different varieties of pre-cooked tinned beans available. Eating them can really benefit your heart, so it is worth experimenting.

Alcohol

This is one of the most controversial areas of the Mediterranean diet. American dietitians and scientists are more likely to recommend that you cut out all alcohol than are their European equivalents, so go with whatever makes you comfortable, remembering that there is some suggestion that a little alcohol can be helpful. Men over 40 and post-menopausal women seem to benefit most from having a little alcohol on a regular basis, but the margin between benefit and harm is comparatively slender. Moderation is definitely essential or the disadvantages are greater than the advantages.

Determining a moderate amount and putting that into practice is not particularly straightforward, however, and we have to rely to some extent on common sense. There are official guidelines, but even those are not easy to follow.

- For a man, a 'safe' upper limit is 3–4 units a day.
- For a woman the upper limit is 2–3 units.
- Both should have two alcohol-free days a week.

The limits for women are lower because they are, on average, smaller and have a different proportion of body fat. The amount that seems to confer benefits in terms of heart disease is actually lower than that, only 1–2 units a day.

A unit of wine is a small glass, 125ml. But strength plays a part and many wines are stronger than they used to be, with alcohol by volume percentages being considerably higher: a 125ml glass of a 12 per cent wine is actually 1.5 units. In addition, the smallest wine glass size is now often 175ml, with some wine bars offering even larger 250ml ones.

Half a pint of beer can be one unit at 3.5 per cent alcohol, but the same quantity of premium beer, at 8–9 per cent, would be 2.5 units. The best advice is to be circumspect and to remember that while alcohol contains no fat, it certainly contains calories, and lots of them. Detailed information can be found in the listings (see page pages 148–50).

Cooking methods

Actually doing some cooking is critical. Relying on ready meals, processed food and takeaways will not do your blood cholesterol levels any good at all, and will have a significant negative impact on many other areas of your health. Your blood pressure, for example, could be seriously affected by the quantity of salt you consume – some shop-bought sandwiches contain as much as seven packets of crisps, for example – and that's without considering the saturated and trans fat content of these foods. If you cut these out of your diet, or reserve them for occasional treats, then you will be making a significant positive change and one that is comparatively simple to implement. Plan your meals, use your freezer and see cooking as a pleasure rather than a chore, and you'll be more than half-way there.

Always think about the way you cook food. The fats you choose are critical, but so are the methods you use. The way you cook a meal can have a profound effect on its nutritional content, increasing calories and adding to the fat load. If you grill bacon on a rack, the fat drains away; if you fry it in a pan with some mushrooms and an egg, it does not. Adding sugar substantially increases calories for no nutritional benefits, and overcooking can cause fibre to break down.

When you boil vegetables, for example, make sure you don't overdo it. Though boiling is good – you're not adding any fats – boiled vegetables lose most of their water-soluble vitamins. They retain more nutrients if they are cooked with a minimum amount of water and for the shortest possible time. Steaming and microwaving retain more, but a significant proportion are still lost, while casseroling food ensures that the vitamins it contains are retained (they are retained in soup, too). You don't need to start a casserole by frying the ingredients, though you can get away with doing that and using only a small quantity of oil if you have good non-stick cooking equipment.

Experiment with methods of cooking other than frying or roasting – such as stir-frying or grilling. If you do fry anything, use only a very little oil and select your oil wisely. Alternatively, you can dry-fry foods that already contain some fat.

Investing in good-quality non-stick pans will help you to cut down on the amount of fat you use, and you may be able to get away with an oil and water spray. At the very least buy yourself a set of small liquid measures, in various gradations of table- and teaspoon sizes. They usually come in a set of one tablespoon (15ml), one teaspoon (5ml), half a teaspoon (2.5ml) and a quarter teaspoon (1.25ml). It is much better to use these accurate measures for oils than either to guess or to use ordinary spoons which can vary in size. Half a teaspoon of oil is the most you should need in a decent non-stick frying pan. If you are trying to lose weight, then it is worth getting some good scales for weighing food.

Finally, don't add breadcrumbs or batter to meat or fish as these extras add calories and soak up fat. Deep-fried vegetables, especially chips, are bad news, and banana fritters should be struck off any heart-friendly menu.

Adapting existing recipes

Everyone has their own particular favourite dishes and there is no reason to stop cooking most of them providing you check them out carefully and make a few adjustments if necessary.

- Reduce the amount of fat and change the type, and cut right back on the salt content.
- Sugar quantities can also often be reduced and dried fruit purée makes a good alternative, especially in cakes.
- Remember to reduce the quantity of cheese if you don't want to substitute a lower-fat variety, and if you make sauces, always use skimmed milk.
- Pulses can be added to casseroles and the quantity of meat reduced.

• Use yoghurt, crème fraîche or fromage frais instead of cream, but low- or half-fat varieties may need to be stabilised first with a little cornflour so they don't separate in cooking.

Food labelling

You don't have to rely on your own knowledge when you are shopping; you can use the information on packaging to help you – but there are some factors to be borne in mind. Most pre-packaged food has a certain amount of information on the packs, ranging from details in the name of the product itself ('light', for example) to detailed nutritional breakdowns. Some of this information is useful, some of it can be misleading, and some of it – such as product names – can be discounted.

Pick up, for example, a packet of oatcakes – basically a healthy item in a cardio-protective diet. The most useful pieces of information on the packaging are the list of ingredients and the nutritional breakdown panel. The ingredients, which are listed in decreasing order of quantity, are: oatmeal, olive oil (9.4 per cent), salt, barley malt extract. The most important thing to note here is that there is no palm oil, a saturated fat that is often found in oatcakes. There is, however, quite a lot of salt.

The nutritional information panel will give a more detailed breakdown. Figures are given both per oatcake and per 100g; the 100g figures make it easier for you to compare like for like across brands and products.

The fats in the oatcakes are broken down into total fat, saturates, mono- and polyunsaturates, and there are 2.9g of saturates in 100g. You can see that some alternative brands on the shelf have more saturates and a lower proportion of monounsaturates.

However, you should also consider the salt content, which is less easily understood. It is marked as sodium, and to get the salt quantity you need to multiply that figure by 2.5. In the case of these particular oatcakes, there are 2g of salt in 100g – but it's not always easy to do the maths in a busy supermarket. Follow broad general guidelines if there's no salt equivalent given: 0.5g of sodium per 100g in anything is a lot; and these oatcakes have 0.8g, so it may be worth checking the other brands again and seeing if you can find a better combination of saturated fat and salt. It's a balancing act, and there is no need to become completely obsessive if you are eating a broadly healthy diet, but the information on packaging can be useful.

You have to be wary about some claims. Ingredients and nutritional information panels are reliable, but other claims are more flexible. There are broad definitions for some, though.

'Fat free' actually means less than 0.15g per 100g of product; 'low fat' means 3g or less and 'reduced fat' products should have 25 per cent less fat than the standard equivalents. This can still mean there is quite a lot of fat, however, especially if the standard version is high in fat – and they can still be high in calories, with calories from fat replaced by calories from sugars. 'Cholesterol free' products can still be high in fat too. The description 'high fibre' applies if there is 6g fibre per 100g of product, or more than 6g in a reasonable daily helping. As a general guideline, 3g of fibre is a lot, 0.5g is a little.

It can be confusing and sometimes it gets worse. Some products have an 'X per cent fat free' tagline. In these cases, remember that something which is 90 per cent fat free still has 10 per cent fat, and check it out in more detail. The recent introduction of 'traffic light' labels has not helped much – there are several different types in operation and they are for varying portion sizes. Don't go by them alone. Once again, common sense must come to the rescue.

SAMPLE MENUS

Here are a few ideas to start you off and inspire you to create your own menus. This is a lifestyle change and not a short-term option, so flexibility is vital. Try to vary what you eat within the basic principles of the Mediterranean diet; there's plenty of room for manoeuvre. And don't forget that you can add your own snacks, so long as they are healthy ones.

Day 1

Breakfast: Muesli with skimmed milk and natural low-fat yoghurt, fruit juice
Lunch: Tomato and red pepper soup, small wholemeal roll; a piece of fruit
Dinner: Roast vegetable cous-cous with grilled chicken; an assortment of melon slices; a square of 70 per cent cocoa-solids chocolate

Day 2

Breakfast: Two slices of wholemeal toast, with olive-oil spread and Marmite
Lunch: Fruit juice; lentil and mushroom soup; a bowl of strawberries with yoghurt
Dinner: Baked salmon with ginger and lemon grass, boiled rice and steamed Oriental vegetables; fresh fruit salad

Day 3

Breakfast: Oat-based cold cereal with chopped banana and skimmed milk; fruit juice
Lunch: Smoked fish pâté with wholemeal toast (no butter necessary), celery and carrot sticks; two plums or satsumas
Dinner: Greek salad, made with feta cheese and lots of tomatoes; low-fat Greek yoghurt with dried fruit, a teaspoon of honey and a few toasted almonds

Day 4

Breakfast: Porridge with skimmed milk; fruit juice
Lunch: Cold chicken and salad sandwich made with wholemeal bread; low-fat yoghurt; a large apple
Dinner: Grilled tuna with seasonal vegetables, brown rice or a baked potato; plum compôte

Day 5

Breakfast: A boiled egg with a slice of wholemeal toast; fruit juice
Lunch: Lentil, yellow pepper and bacon salad; a piece of fresh fruit
Dinner: Mushroom pâté; wholewheat pasta with home-made pesto and a large green salad; baked oranges

EATING OUT

There is no reason to feel that you can't eat out when you are eating for the good of your heart. In general, it is perfectly possible to make heart-friendly choices and find acceptable alternatives on most menus, which is particularly important if you find yourself eating out regularly. The special occasion or celebratory meal can remain a one-off, not something you are going to indulge in often, and you can grant yourself some leeway in those circumstances. However, you really should think about the content of dishes and make sensible choices at other times.

In the following pages there are some general guidelines that can be applied in most restaurants, and then some information that may help you when making a choice from a few specific cuisines, some of which are more compatible with a cardio-protective diet than others.

When you are in a restaurant, think about the basic principles of the Mediterranean diet and choose dishes that contain a lot of vegetables and fruit, whether they are cooked or not – salads are just as valuable as other vegetables. Avoid fatty sauces (including gravy), lots of cheese and don't have huge portions of red meat. Soup usually makes a good starter (unless it's smothered in cream) and you can accompany it with bread – but don't butter the bread and choose wholemeal rather than white if you can. Fruit juice is another useful option.

One tip from the GI diets may help when it comes to main courses: mentally divide your plate into quarters. One quarter should be protein – meat, poultry or fish; one quarter carbs and half vegetables. Try not to have too large a portion of meat; go for one about the size of the back of your clenched fist, or just three slices from a roast. Trim off visible fat or skin and put it to one side. Ask for vegetables to be served without melted butter and salads without dressing; you can always ask for these separately and then add as much or as little as you need. Baked potatoes in their skins are better than roast potatoes, chips or potato wedges, and have more fibre than boiled potatoes. Avoid fried accompaniments, choosing boiled rice rather than a pilau or egg-fried version, for example. If you go for the plainest dishes, the ones with the least elaborate sauces, such as grilled meat or fish, you will be making heart-healthy choices comparatively painlessly.

When it comes to desserts, many restaurants will offer fresh fruit or a fresh fruit salad, though you should avoid adding cream. Ice creams should be an infrequent treat, but sorbets are generally fine and some restaurants now offer granitas. Meringues may be tempting – egg white, no fat – but do remember that they are likely to come with cream, probably lots of it in the case of dishes like Pavlova, and they're full of sugar as well. Finally, have coffee black.

Now for some more specific suggestions.

Chinese

Go for soups as starters rather than fried spring rolls, prawn crackers and the like. Steamed wontons are also worth considering. Avoid deep-fried dishes and choose simple stir-fried ones, which are much lower in fat; best of all are those which are relatively plain and cooked like a stew. The presence of batter is not a good sign, and sweet and sour battered dishes are often served in a high-sugar sauce. Stick to boiled rice and plain boiled noodles.

French

Traditional French restaurants can be a problem, as many dishes are high in fat, cooked and/or served with butter and cream. However this style of cooking is becoming less common and you should be able to find healthier choices on most menus. Salads are often available as starters as well as accompaniments, and soups are an option. Watch out for lavish high-fat sauces with main courses and choose plain dishes or those with simple wine- or vegetable-based sauces instead. Flavoured butters are common with grilled meat or fish, and again these should be avoided – just ask for yours to be served without them. Avoid accompanying vegetables cooked with cream, and make sensible dessert choices too.

Greek, Turkish and Middle-Eastern

Many of these restaurants offer similar dishes and there is almost always some plain grilled meat or fish available. Tsatsiki (yoghurt and cucumber), which may also be called *caçik*, is a good choice of starter but go easy on the flat bread. Filo pastry is common but should be avoided; though it is low in fat by itself, the layers are usually sandwiched together with butter. Stuffed vegetables or vine leaves are often available – generally good – and there might well be a range of pulse dishes (though these could come with a lot of oil). Eat main courses with boiled rice or cous-cous, which can help to fill you up, though grilled kebabs are often served with a salad, which may be enough. Choose fruit for dessert, and note that Turkish coffee is usually served very sweet, often with a few cubes of Turkish delight alongside – think of the calories!

Indian

A lot of Indian food is high in saturated fat, and in fat generally, so be careful. Curries with a strong emphasis on coconut, including kormas, are not a good option, and neither are many deep-fried dishes, like pakoras, samosas and bhajis. Stuffed breads, such as peshwari naan, can be very high in calories so go for plain versions. There are some real advantages to Indian cookery, though, as it puts great emphasis on pulses, particularly lentils and chickpeas, so select dhals and other bean dishes. In North Indian restaurants you can usually find plain meat or fish dishes, tandooris or tikkas, and they are an excellent option, accompanied with boiled rice. Traditional sweets are very high in calories and some are also deep fried; avoid them.

Italian

Many people automatically think about Italian food when they think of Mediterranean cookery, but that doesn't mean that all the food you find in Italian restaurants falls into heart-friendly territory. Garlic bread is packed with butter and there are usually some very rich sauces, often based on cream; choose tomato-based ones for preference. Filled pasta tends to be high in fats, so lasagne and cannelloni are worth avoiding. Fried fish and fried and coated meat escalopes are often found on menus – not, generally, good options – and when it comes to pizza, avoid thick bases and fat-heavy toppings. Italian ice creams are wonderful but high in saturates; opt instead for lower-fat sorbets or desserts made using fresh fruit.

Mexican

It is probably best to treat Mexican food as a rare treat when you are trying to reduce your cholesterol. A lot of it is high in fat and focused on meat, and it can be very difficult to make wise choices. Be wary of tempting nibbles like nachos, dips, and anything made with sour cream or grated cheese; avoid the refried beans and fatty meats. Flour tortillas are higher in fat than those made with corn, but any which have been deep fried are a no-no.

Thai

As with Chinese food, avoid deep-fried dishes. Select clear soups and, in this case, seafood salads. Stir-fries are also generally a good choice but don't go for anything containing coconut cream or milk. Keep rice plain and be careful with dessert selections.

Fast food

If you eat a lot of fast food, one of the best things you can do to reduce your cholesterol immediately is to stop. Cut it right back or keep fast food for a treat if you cannot avoid it completely. Stick with small portion sizes, avoid chips, milkshakes and high-calorie fizzy drinks, going for diet versions of the latter instead. You need to be aware, too, that although some of the fast-food chains have introduced healthier salads, the dressings which accompany them often blow health claims out of the water.

Sandwiches

The best thing you can do for your cholesterol levels is to make your own, so you control the ingredients. Failing that, a sandwich bar that makes them fresh while you wait is probably a better place to buy your sandwich than a chain retailer; recent tests have shown that pre-packed sandwiches can be frighteningly high in fats and salt. In sandwich bars keep your choices simple, avoiding any pre-made mixes or fillings with lots of mayonnaise. Go for sandwiches with plain meat – chicken would be ideal – and salad on wholemeal, and buy fruit rather than a packet of crisps.

...and snacks

When it comes to snacks to see you through the day, bear in mind that many are high in salt or fat, and go for a piece of fresh fruit, a few olives or a handful of dried fruit instead. A low-fat yoghurt is another possibility. If you are getting enough fibre in your diet you may find that you don't need to snack as much anyway, so think about whether you really need a nibble before giving in to habit or temptation.

HOW TO USE THIS BOOK

All the foods and drinks in these listings are grouped into categories, and each category begins with some general guidelines on making the best choices. The items themselves are listed down the left-hand side of each page, followed by information about how much and what type of fat they contain. In some categories you will find figures for the fat content of specific dishes; these are for basic recipes and are intended as a general guideline.

It would be almost impossible to eliminate saturated fat from your diet completely; remember that sources of mono- and polyunsaturated fats will contain some saturates as well. The key is eating saturates in proportion to other fats. You need to minimise the saturated fat element, and the figures given in the listings can help. There is no need to calculate exactly every single gram of saturated fat you take in but you need enough information to make sensible choices – and here it is.

Remember that cholesterol is confined to products of animal origin (this can be difficult to establish with some processed foods and apparently unlikely items, though). People with high blood cholesterol levels used to be advised to avoid those foods that were particularly high in it – eggs, some seafood, offal. Now the advice is either to eat them in moderation, limiting servings to three times a week, or not to worry over much as dietary cholesterol does not seem to be a significant factor in the overall level of cholesterol in the blood. If your diet is lower in fat, it is almost inevitably going to be lower in cholesterol anyway. In some circumstances you may be advised to take a more rigorous approach, for example if you have a particular blood disorder. If this applies to you, it is highly likely that your doctor will already have spoken to you about it.

Throughout the listings, most figures given are per 100g or 100ml of the food in question so comparison is easy, with no distractions about comparing portion sizes and no need to do elaborate maths before you can look at one food in relation to another. Do consider portion sizes, though, when it comes to what you actually eat and reduce them if necessary, especially if you are trying to lose weight. A hundred grams of chips may not look too bad in terms of fat –

but 100g of chips is only about 10-12 chip shop ones: you are likely to eat a much bigger portion than that.

For total fat, saturated fat, mono- and poly-unsaturated fats, the figures are for the quantity in grams found in 100g of the food under consideration. Because cholesterol is present in much smaller quantities relative to fat, it is given in milligrams per 100g. There are also figures for calorie content per 100g or 100ml. In two categories almost all of the items listed contain no fat but can have a considerable impact in terms of calories – alcoholic drinks and sugar – so don't be tempted into thinking they are fine because they're fat-free.

COLUMNS IN THE LISTINGS – SUMMARY

The first column gives the total fat content of each item in grams. The second gives the amount of saturated fat and the two following ones are for mono- and polyunsaturates. The fifth column is the cholesterol. Some of the totals will not add up to the total amount of fat because other kinds of fatty acids are also present in much smaller quantities, but these do not affect the basic balance. The very last column is the calories.

In the fast-moving food industry, new products are launched all the time while old ones slip out of circulation and existing ones are modified, sometimes to take into account recommendations on public health.

Ready meals and processed foods are also changing, both in their scope and in their basic recipes, and manufacturers usually provide some level of nutritional information on the packaging. This may be comprehensive, with total fats broken down into saturates, monounsaturates and polyunsaturates, and even with omega-3s and cholesterol on occasion. It may also be comparatively sketchy, with perhaps just a total fat figure. Use this information to guide your choices, making sure you check the main nutritional information panel in cases where figures are found in more than one place, and always go by the 100g figures as portion sizes vary enormously.

The *Collins Gem Calorie Counter* may also be of help. It includes a lot of branded foods, and has a total fat grams per 100g figure for each one, though the fats are not broken down into types. The extra calorie figures are invaluable if you are trying to lose weight as well as reduce the amount and proportion of potentially damaging fats in your diet.

Values for unbranded foods have been obtained from McCance and Widdowson, The Composition of Foods (6th summary edition, 2002), and have been reproduced by permission of the Controller of Her Majesty's Stationery Office. Recipe breakdowns for the basic dishes can also be found there. Asda have also kindly supplied information for some of their own-brand lines, and other information has come from manufacturers and retailers, to whom the publishers are grateful.

CONVERSION CHART

Metric to imperial

100 grams (g) = 3.53 ounces (oz)
1 kilogram (kg) = 2.2 pounds (lb)
100 millilitres (ml) = 3.38 fluid ounces (fl oz)
1 litre = 1.76 pints

Imperial to metric

1 ounce (oz) = 28.35 grams (g)
1 pound (lb) = 453.60 grams (g)
1 stone (st) = 6.35 kilograms (kg)
1 fluid ounce (fl oz) = 29.57 millilitres (ml)
1 pint = 0.568 litres (l)

ABBREVIATIONS USED IN THE LISTINGS

Sat	saturated fat
Mono	monounsaturated
Poly	polyunsaturated
Chol	cholesterol
Cal	calories
g	gram
mg	milligram
kcal	calorie
N	no specific figures are available, but the product contains a significant amount
n/k	not known
tr	trace
e	estimate

BAKERY

Bread can make a valuable contribution to the diet, but be careful to keep to loaves made – as far as possible – from wholegrains, as the fibre they contain is important for the digestive system as well as cholesterol levels. Wholegrain flour also contains more nutrients than white refined flours, especially B vitamins. Refined-flour products are less satisfying and choosing wholemeal options can keep you feeling full for longer, which is useful if you're trying to lose weight. Cakes are best avoided as they are almost uniformly high in calories and many contain trans fats. If you can't resist them completely, only have small portions and choose ones without fatty fillings or icing.

TIP: Making your own bread can be quick and easy, especially if you use easy-bake or quick yeast. Follow a straightforward recipe (some packs of yeast have good basic ones) and knead the dough in the bowl; there's no need to take over the entire kitchen. Put it into tins, allow to rise for 30 minutes and then bake according to the instructions. Use good flour and you'll really notice the difference between your own bread and industrially produced loaves.

Food type	Total fat (g)	Sat (g)	Mono (g)	Poly (g)	Chol (mg)	Cal (kcal)
Breads						
Brown bread	2	0.4	0.4	0.7	0	207
Chapati, made with fat	12.8	N	N	N	N	328
Chapati, made without fat	1	0.1	0.1	0.4	0	202
Ciabatta	3.9	0.6	2.1	0.9	tr	271
Ciabatta, luxury	5.9	0.6	3.9	1	tr	275
Cracked wheat bread	3.9	0.9	1.9	0.7	n/k	240
Currant loaf	7.6	1.6e	1.5e	2e	0	289
'Danish style' white bread	2.7	0.5e	0.5e	0.9e	0	228
Farmhouse loaf, white	2	0.5	0.4	0.6	0	236
French stick, white	1.9	0.3	0.3	0.7	0	263
Garlic bread, prepacked, frozen, part baked	18.3	9.7	5.5	1.5	37	365
Granary bread	2.3	0.6	0.6	0.8	0	237
Naan bread, including garlic and coriander	7.3	1	3.1	2.4	5	285
New York Deli bread, Terence Stamp	1.4	0.3	0.2	0.7	n/k	184
Pitta bread, white	1.3	0.2	0.1	0.5	0	255
Pitta bread, wholemeal	2.3	0.5	0.9	0.8	0	225

TIP: Choosing – or baking – bread with added seeds is a good way of adding these to your diet. Watch out for seeded loaves or add roughly ground linseeds, sunflower and pumpkin seeds to the dry ingredients of breadmaking before you add the liquid.

Food type	Total fat (g)	Sat (g)	Mono (g)	Poly (g)	Chol (mg)	Cal (kcal)
Pitta bread, wholemeal, organic	1	0.2	n/k	n/k	0	210
Poppadoms	38.8	8	16.5	12.5	2	501
Rye bread	1.7	0.3	0.3	0.3	0	219
Rye and sunflower seed, Mestenacher	3.6	0.6	N	N	0	191
Soda bread	3	0.5	1.5	1	n/k	208
Wheatgerm bread	3.1	0.7	0.7	1.1	0	220
White bread, sliced	1.6	0.3	0.3	0.5	0	219
White bread, premium	2.3	N	N	N	N	230
White bread, fried in lard	32.2	12.5	13.4	2.9	tr	498
White bread, toasted	2	0.4	0.4	0.6	tr	267
White bread with added fibre	1.5	0.4	0.6	0.3	0	230
White bread with added fibre, toasted	1.8	0.5	0.7	0.3	0	273
Wholemeal bread	2.5	0.5	0.6	0.8	0	217
Wholemeal bread, stoneground	2.3	0.8	N	N	0	217
Wholemeal bread, toasted	2.9	0.5	0.7	1	0	255
Rolls, etc						
Bagels, plain	1.8	N	N	N	0	273

TIP: Wholemeal bread is not the same as brown bread. Brown bread has had some of the bran removed, it only uses 85 per cent of the grain and may have caramelising sweeteners added. Wholemeal bread, also called wholegrain, uses 100 per cent of the grain and contains insoluble fibre, good for the digestive system, and several other nutrients.

Food type	Total fat (g)	Sat (g)	Mono (g)	Poly (g)	Chol (mg)	Cal (kcal)
Bagels, cinnamon and raisin	2	0.3	N	N	0	253
Bagels, onion	3.1	0.5	N	N	0	255
Breadsticks	8.4	5.9	1.3	0.9	0	392
Brown rolls, crusty	2.8	0.6	0.6	0.7	0	255
Brown rolls, soft	3.2	1.1	1	1	0	236
Croissants	19.7	9.8	4.6	1.6	52	373
Croissants, luxury, average	21.6	13.3	6.2	0.7	n/k	400
Granary rolls	4.2	1.1e	1.1e	1.4e	0	238
Hamburger buns	5	1.1	1.3	1.1	0	264
Rice cakes	3.6	N	N	N	N	374
Taco shells	26	N	N	N	0	506
Tortilla wraps	7.8	2.8	N	N	0	306
Tortillas, corn	7	N	N	N	0	343
Tortillas, flour	11.7	N	N	N	0	323
White rolls, crusty	2.2	0.5	0.5	0.7	0	262
White rolls, soft	2.6	0.6	0.6	0.8	0	254
Wholemeal rolls	3.3	0.8	0.9	0.7	0	244
Buns and pastries						
Chelsea buns	14.2	3	4.5	5.9	33	368
Crumpets, toasted	1	0.1	0.1	0.5	0	207
Currant buns	5.6	1.9	2	1.2	2	280
Custard tarts, individual	14.5	6.1	6	1.4	95	277
Danish pastries, average	14.1	8.6	2	1.9	41	342
Doughnuts, jam	14.5	4.3	5.4	3.6	15	336
Doughnuts, ring	22.4	5.8	9.4	6.1	24	403

Food type	Total fat (g)	Sat (g)	Mono (g)	Poly (g)	Chol (mg)	Cal (kcal)
Eccles cake	17.8	N	N	N	13	387
Hot cross buns	7	1.8	2.1	2.5	23	312
Jam tarts, average	14.7	6.6	5.1	1.8	42	383
Mince pies	21.3	N	N	N	12	435
Muffins, English style, white	1.9	0.4	0.5	0.6	0	223
Muffins, English style, white, toasted	2.7	0.4	0.5	0.7	0	261
Muffins, US style, blueberry	17.1	1.7	10.1	4.4	n/k	340
Muffins, US style, chocolate chip	18.2	10.7	5.2	0.9	68	385
Scones, fruit	8.7	2.4	4.1	1.7	6	315
Scones, plain	14.8	3.7	4.5	5.9	6	364
Scones, wholemeal	14.6	3.6	4.4	5.8	6	328
Scotch pancakes	9.6	0.7	3.5	2.1	21	270
Teacakes, toasted	8.3	2.9	2.7	1.5	20	329
Cakes and cream cakes						
Almond slice	26	8.3	11.2	5.9	10	426
Banana bread	13.6	2.4	3.9	6.5	33	338
Battenburg cake	16.8	3.4	6	6.4	74	373
Cake mix, made up following instructions	11.6	6	4.3	0.8	67	322
Caramel shortcake	32.2	20.7	6.9	3	n/k	525
Carrot cake, with topping	22.7	5.5	5.3	10.7	42	359
Chocolate éclair	29.4	15.3	10.7	2.1	n/k	400
Chocolate fudge cake	14.3	4.6	6.4	2.7	17	358
Chocolate mini roll	25.1	15.9	7.9	1.3	n/k	443

Food type	Total fat (g)	Sat (g)	Mono (g)	Poly (g)	Chol (mg)	Cal (kcal)
Crispie cakes, made with plain chocolate	18	10.7	5.7	0.8	4	461
Eclairs, frozen	30.6	16.1	10.2	1.9	150	396
Fancy iced cakes, including fondant fancies	9.1	N	N	N	N	355
Fruit cake, plain, sultana	14.8	6.9	5.9	1.2	N	371
Fruit cake, rich	11.4	2.4	3.7	4.5	46	343
Fruit cake, rich, coated with royal icing and marzipan	9.8	1.8	3.8	3.6	31	350
Fruit cake, wholemeal	16.2	3.5	5.1	6.5	50	366
Gateau, frozen, chocolate based	15.7	9	3.8	1.2	56	295
Gateau, frozen, fruit	12.3	7	2.9	0.9	53	248
Greek pastries, average, including baklava	17	N	N	N	N	322
Madeira cake	15.1	8.4	3.8	1.6	N	377
Malt loaf, fruit	2.3	0.5	1	1	0	295
Reduced-fat cake	4.2	1.5	1.3	0.6	8	281
Sponge cake	27.2	5.8	8.9	10.9	112	467
Sponge cake, 'fat free'	6.9	1.9	2.6	1.2	227	301
Sponge cake, jam filled, including Swiss roll	4.9	1.6	1.7	0.7	N	302
Sponge cake, frozen, with dairy cream and jam	10.9	N	N	N	59	280
Swiss rolls, individual, chocolate	16.8	7	7.2	1.5	86	386
Trifle sponges	3.7	1.1	N	N	n/k	324

BAKING PRODUCTS

Choose wholemeal flour for baking and be extremely careful about the fat you use (see Understanding and choosing fats, pages 37-46). Bear in mind that many baking ingredients – such as marzipan or sugar – are high in calories even if they are low in fat. Pastry, high in both calories and saturated fat, is best avoided but if you need to use it there are some tricks you can use. Filo pastry, for instance, usually has melted butter brushed between each sheet. Make this a healthier option by using olive oil instead for savoury dishes, and comparatively tasteless rapeseed oil in sweet ones.

TIP: Reduce the amount of sugar used in cooking. Many recipes will be fine with less, or you can use a dried fruit purée instead.

Food type	Total fat (g)	Sat (g)	Mono (g)	Poly (g)	Chol (mg)	Cal (kcal)
Barley flour	1.7	n/k	n/k	n/k	0	360
Bran, wheat	5.5	0.9	0.7	2.9	0	206
Buckwheat flour	1.5	0	n/k	n/k	0	364
Chapati flour, white	0.5	0.1	tr	0.2	0	333
Chapati flour, brown	1.2	0.2	0.1	0.5	0	335
Cornflour	0.7	0.1	0.1	0.3	0	354
Gram flour (chickpea flour)	5.4e	0.5e	1.1e	2.7e	0	313
Granary flour (malted brown)	2.1	0.4	n/k	n/k	0	334
Pasta flour	1.9	0.4	n/k	n/k	0	327
Rye flour	2	0.3	0.2	0.9	0	335
Soya flour, full fat	23.5	2.9	4.5	11.4	0	447
Soya flour, low fat	7.2	0.9	1.4	3.5	0	352
Spelt flour	2.4	0.3	n/k	n/k	0	311
Wheat flour, white, plain	1.3	0.2	0.1	0.6	0	341
Wheat flour, white, self-raising	1.2	0.2	0.1	0.5	0	330
Wheat flour, white, 'strong' or breadmaking	1.4	0.2	0.1	0.6	0	341
Wheat flour, brown	2	0.3	0.2	0.9	0	324
Wheat flour, brown malted, with sunflower seeds	2.8	0.7	n/k	n/k	0	351
Wheat flour, wholemeal	2.2	0.3	0.3	1	0	310

TIP: When baking, either use non-stick tins that you don't have to grease or line them with non-stick greaseproof paper (and grease that only lightly).

Food type	Total fat (g)	Sat (g)	Mono (g)	Poly (g)	Chol (mg)	Cal (kcal)
Wheatgerm	9.2	1.3	1.1	4.2	0	357
Bread mixes						
Parmesan and sun-dried tomato bread mix	1.7	0.5	n/k	n/k	n/k	229
Sunflower bread mix	6.3	0.9	n/k	n/k	0	259
White bread mix	1.8	0.4	n/k	n/k	0	245
Wholemeal bread mix	2.2	0.6	n/k	n/k	0	210
Baking ingredients						
Baking powder	0	0	0	0	0	163
Marzipan, home-made, with egg	25.8	2.2	17.4	4.8	29	462
Marzipan, white and yellow, retail	12.7	1	8	3.1	0	389
Mixed peel	0.9	N	N	N	0	231
Mincemeat	4.3	N	N	N	4	274
Yeast, compressed	0.4	N	N	N	0	53
Yeast, dried	1.5	N	N	N	0	169
Pastry						
Filo pastry, raw weight	2.7	0.3	N	N	N	234
Flaky pastry, raw weight	31.1	9.7	11.8	8	16	427

TIP: If you find it difficult to tolerate wheat, try using spelt flour instead; many people find it more acceptable. You can use it in baking, breadmaking (it rises more quickly, though) and spelt-based products – like spelt pasta – are becoming more widely available.

Food type	Total fat (g)	Sat (g)	Mono (g)	Poly (g)	Chol (mg)	Cal (kcal)
Flaky pastry, cooked	41	12.8	15.6	10.5	21	564
Puff pastry	27.7	15	N	N	n/k	400
Shortcrust pastry, raw weight	28.1	8.7	10.6	7.3	14	451
Shortcrust pastry, cooked	32.6	10.1	12.3	8.4	17	524
Wholemeal pastry, raw weight	28.7	8.8	10.7	7.5	14	433
Wholemeal pastry, cooked	33.2	10.2	12.4	8.7	17	501

TIP: Most commercially made baked products are high in saturated fats, and frequently in trans fats too. They are also often high in sugars, so be cautious.

BEANS, PULSES AND CEREALS

Beans, pulses and some cereals – oats, rye and barley – are particularly high in soluble fibre, which makes you feel full up. Postponing the onset of hunger isn't fibre's only benefit, though: eating more soluble fibre can help to reduce cholesterol levels. Try to incorporate pulses in your diet on a regular basis, perhaps using them to replace some of the meat in casseroles or adding them to salads. If you prepare beans properly, throwing out the soaking water and cooking them in fresh, and if you eat them regularly, you should not suffer any digestive discomfort.

TIP: Many cooked pulses make delicious salads, and their texture contrasts nicely with crisp, crunchy vegetables like celery and chopped peppers. Dress bean and lentil salads when the pulses are still warm, and keep the dressing quite sharp.

Food type	Total fat (g)	Sat (g)	Mono (g)	Poly (g)	Chol (mg)	Cal (kcal)
Beans and pulses						
Aduki beans, dried and boiled	0.2	N	N	N	0	123
Baked beans in tomato sauce	0.6	0.1	0.1	0.3	0	84
Baked beans, reduced sugar and salt	0.6	0.1	0.1	0.3	0	73
Baked beans in tomato sauce with pork sausages	3.3	1.2	N	N	n/k	93
Blackeye beans, dried	1.6	0.5	0.1	0.7	0	311
Blackeye beans, boiled	0.6	0.5	0.1	0.7	0	116
Black turtle beans, dried	0.9	0.2	n/k	n/k	0	350
Borlotti beans, canned, drained	0.4	0.1	n/k	n/k	0	103
Butter beans, canned, drained and reheated	0.5	0.1	tr	0.2	0	77
Cannellini beans, canned, drained	0.3	0.1	n/k	n/k	0	84
Chickpeas, dried	5.4	0.5	1.1	2.7	0	320
Chickpeas, dried, boiled	2.1	0.2	0.4	1	0	121
Chickpeas, canned, drained and reheated	2.9	0.3	0.7	1.3	0	115
Flageolet beans, canned and drained	1.1	0.2	n/k	n/k	0	72

TIP: Some pulses – notably kidney beans and their relatives such as cannellini beans – need to be boiled sharply at the start of cooking. Then simmer them until they are tender.

Food type	Total fat (g)	Sat (g)	Mono (g)	Poly (g)	Chol (mg)	Cal (kcal)
Haricot beans, canned and drained	0.3	tr	n/k	n/k	0	69
Lentils, green/brown, dried	1.9	0.2	0.3	0.8	0	297
Lentils, green/brown, dried, boiled	0.7	0.1	0.1	0.3	0	105
Lentils, red, dried	1.3	0.2	0.2	0.5	0	318
Lentils, red, boiled	0.4	tr	0.1	0.2	0	100
Mung beans, dried	1.1	0.3	0.1	0.5	0	279
Mung beans, boiled	0.4	0.3	0.1	0.5	0	91
Pinto beans, canned, drained	0.7	0.3	n/k	n/k	0	102
Red kidney beans, dried	1.4	0.2	0.1	0.8	0	266
Red kidney beans, dried, boiled	0.5	0.2	0.1	0.8	0	103
Red kidney beans, canned, drained and reheated	0.6	0.1	0.1	0.3	0	100
Soya beans, dried	18.6	2.3	3.5	9.1	0	370
Soya beans, boiled	7.3	0.9	1.4	3.5	0	141
Tofu, steamed	4.2	0.5	0.8	2	0	73
Tofu, steamed and fried	17.7	N	N	N	0	261
Hummus						
Hummus, Tesco	26.8	2.8	14.2	8.5	0	315

TIP: Make sure beans are cooked. Test this by squeezing one between finger and thumb; it should be completely soft. Test larger beans by biting, as these can feel soft on the outside while the inside is still a bit hard.

Food type	Total fat (g)	Sat (g)	Mono (g)	Poly (g)	Chol (mg)	Cal (kcal)
Hummus, 'healthy living', Tesco	11.1	1.3	5.1	4.5	0	184
Hummus, olive and sun-dried tomato, Tesco	25	2.7	13.1	8.2	0	280
Cereals						
Bulgur wheat, dry weight	1.7	0.2	n/k	n/k	0	357
Cous-cous, dry weight	0.6	0.1	0.1	0.2	0	355
Millet seeds, dry weight	4.2	0.7	N	N	0	375
Polenta, dry weight	0.5	n/k	n/k	n/k	0	72
Quinoa, dry weight	5	0.5	1.4	2.1	0	325
Wheat bran	5.5	0.9	0.7	2.9	0	206
For fresh beans, see *Vegetables*						
For flours, see *Baking Products*						

TIP: Add fish to a bean salad. Flake a little smoked mackerel and mix it with cooked mixed beans and thin slices of raw red onion. Sprinkle lemon juice over the salad and mix well. Spoon it onto a bed of chopped cos lettuce and lightly drizzle with olive oil.

BISCUITS, CRACKERS AND CRISPBREADS

Most biscuits are high in fat, often in saturated fats – some still contain quite high levels of trans fats – and may be high in salt (even sweet biscuits). It's also quite hard to stop at one so they are generally best avoided all together. When it comes to savoury crackers, opt for oatcakes as their fibre content can be useful, but do check nutritional panels and compare brands as the balance of fats can differ quite widely. Cream crackers, water biscuits and matzo crackers are all healthy options, and matzo crackers are particularly low in fat.

TIP: Don't see cereal bars as a healthy alternative to cakes, biscuits or confectionery. Not only are they often high in sugar, they are frequently high in fat – and consequently in calories – too. Read the labels, as you sometimes find some surprisingly unhealthy ingredients in what appear to be healthy products.

Food type	Total fat (g)	Sat (g)	Mono (g)	Poly (g)	Chol (mg)	Cal (kcal)
Sweet biscuits						
Amaretti	8.3	N	N	N	n/k	430
Chocolate biscuit bars, fully coated	24.3	13.2	8.4	1.5	22e	501
Chocolate biscuit bars, fully coated, with filling	28.4	16.3	9.2	1.6	11	496
Chocolate chip cookies	22.9	10.6	8.6	2.6	1	474
Chocolate fingers, Cadbury	27.1	10.8	N	N	n/k	515
Crunch creams	24.6	15	6.8	1.7	3	497
Custard creams, Tesco	22.7	11.8	7.4	2.1	n/k	500
Digestive biscuits, plain	20.3	9	8.3	2	41	465
Digestive biscuits, chocolate	24.1	12.2	8.9	1.6	51	493
Flapjacks	27	4.9	7.6	10.3	1	493
Gingernuts	13	6	5.1	1.3	N	436
Jaffa cakes	8.1	4.2	2.8	0.9	47	377
Malted milk, Tesco	21.8	10	8.1	2.3	n/k	490
Milk chocolate 'Take a break', Asda	29.4	18.5	8.8	1	26	526
Nice creams, Tesco	24.4	13.5	7.2	2	n/k	505
Oat-based biscuits, e.g. Hob Nobs, average	21.4	9.2	8.3	2.5	N	468
Rich Tea biscuits	15.2	6	6.3	2.6	n/k	453
Sandwich biscuits, jam filled	17.3	7.2	7.4	1.9	N	439
Sandwich biscuits, cream filled	20.7	11	7.3	1.9	51e	482

Food type	Total fat (g)	Sat (g)	Mono (g)	Poly (g)	Chol (mg)	Cal (kcal)
Semi-sweet biscuits	13.3	6.3	5.1	1.3	31e	427
Short sweet biscuits, such as Shortcake	21.8	11.1	8.1	1.5	37e	454
Shortbread	27.5	18.2	6.7	1.3	74e	509
Wafer biscuits, filled	30.1	20.7	6.8	1	N	537
Wafer bars, chocolate, fully coated	29.7	18.2	9	1	14	513
Savoury biscuits and crackers						
Cheddars	27.7	2.7	N	N	n/k	509
Cream crackers	13.3	5.4	5.8	1.5	N	414
Crispbread, rye	0.6	tr	0.1	0.2	0	308
Crispbread, dark rye	1.7	0.4	N	N	0	308
Crispbread, Ryvita 'original'	1.7	0.3	N	N	0	317
Crispbread, Ryvita, pumpkin seeds and oats	9.9	1.9	3.1	4.5	0	362
Crispbread, multigrain	5.2	0.9	N	N	0	332
Matzo crackers	1.1	0.3	n/k	n/k	0	369
Oatcakes, olive oil, Paterson	17.2	2.9	10.5	3.7	0	412
Oatcakes, rough, Paterson	17.2	2.9	10.5	3.7	0	431

TIP: Experiment with making your own healthy biscuits – if you need motivation, check out the nutritional information on some commercial brands. There are plenty of simple recipes about, and bear in mind that you can often either knock back the quantity of fat, or substitute a dried fruit purée and reduce the sugar too.

Food type	Total fat (g)	Sat (g)	Mono (g)	Poly (g)	Chol (mg)	Cal (kcal)
Water biscuits	12.5	N	N	N	N	440
Wholemeal crackers	11.5	2.3	3.4	5	N	414
For cereal bars, see under *Breakfast cereals* or *Snacks*						

TIP: Think before you spread butter on savoury biscuits and crackers; they don't always need it. Try a little low-fat cream cheese instead, or even Marmite, if you find them too dry.

BREAKFAST CEREALS AND CEREAL BARS

Eating cereal is a good way to begin the day, particularly if it's porridge or muesli. Oats are the best option because they contain soluble fibre, which binds dietary cholesterol and some of the cholesterol-containing bile salts, preventing them being re-absorbed by the liver. But what you add is important too: full-cream milk or 'breakfast' milk can add a lot of fat. Wean yourself off rich milk and get down to skimmed, or try low-fat yoghurt as an alternative. Scatter with chopped dried fruit and you won't miss the milky taste too much – and you'll be adding more fibre as well as having one of your daily portions of fruit. Cereal bars are often high in fat and in saturates – read the nutritional information on the packaging before buying them.

TIP: To maximise the beneficial effects of porridge, add some extra oat bran. The beta-glucan oats contain helps lower cholesterol levels, keeps your blood-sugar levels even and maintains the health of your bowels. Rolled oats have 4g of beta-glucan per 100g serving, and oat bran 5.5 – every little helps.

Food type	Total fat (g)	Sat (g)	Mono (g)	Poly (g)	Chol (mg)	Cal (kcal)
All Bran	4	0.7	0.5	2	0	270
Bran Flakes	2.5	0.4	0.3	1.5	0	330
Cheerios	3.9	1.1	N	N	0	368
Cheerios, honey nut	3.7	0.9	N	N	0	374
Cinnamon Grahams	9.8	3.7	N	N	0	411
Clusters	8.5	2.7	N	N	0	387
Coco Pops	2.5	1	0.6	0.5	0	383
Cookie Crisp	3.4	1.1	N	N	0	378
Clusters	4.8	1.5	N	N	0	387
Cornflakes	0.9	0.2	0.2	0.4	0	376
Crunchy Nut Corn Flakes	3.5	0.7	1.5	1	0	405
Fitnesse	1.3	0.4	N	N	0	373
Frosties	0.6	0.1	0.1	0.4	0	381
Golden Nuggets	1.1	0.3	N	N	0	379
Fruit 'n' Fibre	5	2.5	1	0.7	0	353
Grape Nuts	2	0.4	N	N	0	345
Muesli, Swiss-style	5.9	0.8	2.8	1.6	tr	363
Muesli, Swiss-style, no added sugar	7.8	1.5	3.5	2.4	tr	366
Nesquik cereal	4.1	1.6	N	N	0	381
Nutri-Grain	8.4	1.6	3.3	0.9	tr	360

TIP: Blackberries are high in vitamins C and E, but don't just use them in puddings. Like all berries they make a good snack, and are also delicious scattered over muesli at breakfast.

Food type	Total fat (g)	Sat (g)	Mono (g)	Poly (g)	Chol (mg)	Cal (kcal)
Oat Bran Flakes, with raisins	5	0.8	1.8	2	0	346
Oatibix	8	1.3	N	N	0	377
Oatiflakes	5.6	0.9	N	N	0	381
Oatmeal, quick-cook, raw	9.2	1.6	3.3	3.7	0	357
Oats and More, honey	4.8	0.7	N	N	0	379
Oats and More, almond	8.8	1	N	N	0	398
Optivita, berry	7	1	N	N	0	371
Optivita, raisin	7	1	N	N	0	369
Porridge, made with water	1.1	0.2	0.4	0.5	0	46
Porridge, made with full-cream milk	5.1	2.8	1.5	0.6	14	113
Puffed wheat	1.3	0.2	0.2	0.6	0	321
Ready Brek	8.3	2	3	3.3	0	366
Rice Krispies	1	0.3	0.2	0.4	0	382
Ricicles	0.7	0.2	0.1	0.2	0	378
Shredded Wheat	2.5	0.5	0.3	1	0	332
Shreddies	1.9	0.4	0.3	0.9	0	346
Special K	1	0.3	0.2	0.4	0	376
Sugar Puffs	1	0.2	0.1	0.4	0	381
Sultana Bran	2	0.4	0.2	1	0	316
Weetabix	2.7	0.6	0.3	1.8	0	352

TIP: For a delicious breakfast, serve low-fat Greek yoghurt scattered with blueberries and a few chopped walnuts. Drizzle honey over the top.

Food type	Total fat (g)	Sat (g)	Mono (g)	Poly (g)	Chol (mg)	Cal (kcal)
Cereal Bars						
Cereal chewy bar, average	16.4	5	8.7	1.8	N	419
Cereal crunchy bar, average	22.2	4.5	11.3	5.4	tr	468
Apple and blackcurrant, light, Sainsbury	2.6	0.4	N	N	n/k	286
Apricot, organic, Sainsbury	15	3.5	7.5	3	n/k	421
Cheerios	13.5	8	N	N	n/k	416
Cheerios, honey nut	12.7	7.7	N	N	n/k	406
Cookie Crisp	13.7	8.4	N	N	n/k	417
Crunchy Nut nuts, Kellogs	34	5	N	N	n/k	530
Fitnesse, chocolate	7	3.9	N	N	n/k	382
Fitnesse, chocolate and raspberry	5.7	3	N	N	n/k	375
Fitnesse, chocolate and orange	5.2	2.7	N	N	n/k	377
Fitnesse, original multigrain	6.8	3.2	N	N	n/k	382
Fitnesse, strawberry	7	3.2	N	N	n/k	383
Fruit and fibre wholegrain, Sainsbury	11.1	5.1	2.3	2.9	n/k	405
Multigrain, Jordans	2.4	0.5	1.2	0.7	n/k	364
Nesquik bar	14.9	10.1	N	N	n/k	433
Shreddies	10.4	7.8	N	N	n/k	399
Special K chocolate chip	7	4	N	N	n/k	401
Special K original	8	3.5	N	N	n/k	402

TIP: Try grating a little nutmeg over your porridge just before serving.

CONDIMENTS, SAUCES AND GRAVY

Be circumspect about ready-made sauces, pickles and cook-in sauces. They may not necessarily be high in fat but they often have high sugar levels, raising their calorie content. Salt levels need to be considered in a cardio-protective diet, so check those carefully too. Some stock cubes, for instance, can be very high in salt. Adapt your cooking, flavour your food using other ingredients – herbs and spices can be liberally employed – and avoid ready-made sauces as much as possible. Control the contents of your meals yourself by making your own – but avoid making gravy using all the fat from a roast.

TIP: This comparatively low-fat vinaigrette dressing will dress enough salad for 4–6 people. Put 2 tablespoons of extra virgin olive oil in a clean jar with a lid. Add a tablespoon of white wine vinegar, the juice of a lemon, one teaspoon of Dijon mustard, some fresh thyme leaves and some ground black pepper. Fasten the lid on well and shake the jar vigorously. Increase the quantity of mustard for a stronger taste.

Food type	Total fat (g)	Sat (g)	Mono (g)	Poly (g)	Chol (mg)	Cal (kcal)
Table sauces, dressings and pickles						
Apple chutney, average	0.2	tr	tr	0.1	0	190
Barbecue sauce	0.1	0	0	0.1	0	93
Blue cheese dressing	46.3	N	N	N	41	457
Brinjal (aubergine) pickle	24.4	1.7	n/k	n/k	n/k	367
Brown sauce	0.1	tr	tr	tr	0	98
Caesar salad dressing, average	32	5.1	N	N	n/k	335
French dressing	49.4	8	10.6	28.4	0	462
French dressing, 'fat free'	tr	tr	tr	tr	0	38
Horseradish sauce, average	8.4	1.1	3.8	3.2	14	153
Mango chutney	10.9	N	N	N	0	285
Mayonnaise, shop	75.6	11.4	18.2	42.4	75	691
Mayonnaise, reduced calorie	28.1	4.2	6.9	15.7	22	288
Mayonnaise, Hellmann's, Light	29.8	2.7	N	N	n/k	297
Mayonnaise, Hellmann's, Extra Light	5	0.5	N	N	n/k	88
Mint sauce	tr	tr	tr	tr	0	101

TIP: Try buying spices in relevant stores – typically Indian spices like cumin in an Indian shop, for instance – rather than in supermarkets; the prices will generally be lower by weight. Store them in airtight containers and keep in a dark place like a cupboard, and they should be fine for some time. If they begin to lose their distinctive aroma, smelling musty instead, replace them.

Food type	Total fat (g)	Sat (g)	Mono (g)	Poly (g)	Chol (mg)	Cal (kcal)
Mustard, smooth	8.2	0.5	5.8	1.6	0	139
Mustard, wholegrain	10.2	0.6	7.2	1.9	0	140
Nam Pla (Thai fish sauce)	0.1	0	n/k	n/k	n/k	145
Pesto, classic, Sacla	44.3	6.5	N	N	n/k	438
Pesto, sun-dried tomato, Sacla	27.9	3.9	N	N	n/k	289
Pickle, sweet	0.1	tr	tr	tr	0	141
Piccalilli	0.5	0.1	0.1	0.3	0	84
Relish, burger, chilli / tomato	0.1	tr	tr	tr	0	114
Relish, burger, corn / cucumber / onion	0.3	tr	0.1	0.2	0	119
Salad cream	31	3.3	11.4	14.5	43	348
Salad cream, reduced calorie	17.2	2.5	4.7	9.1	7	194
Soy sauce	tr	0	0	0	0	43
Shoyu soy sauce	0.2	0.2	0	0	0	83
Tamari soy sauce	0.5	0.5	0	0	0	132
Tartare sauce	24.6	N	N	N	49	299
Thousand Island dressing	30.2	N	N	N	29	323
Tomato chutney	0.2	tr	tr	0.1	0	128
Tomato ketchup	0.1	tr	tr	tr	0	115
Worcestershire sauce	0.1	tr	tr	tr	0	65
Cooking sauces, savoury						
Bread sauce, made with whole milk	4	1.9	1.1	0.6	10	110
Bread sauce, made with semi-skimmed milk	2.5	1	0.6	0.5	4	97

Food type	Total fat (g)	Sat (g)	Mono (g)	Poly (g)	Chol (mg)	Cal (kcal)
Cheese sauce, made with whole milk	14.8	7.2	4.2	2.5	30	198
Cheese sauce, made with semi-skimmed milk	12.8	5.9	3.7	2.4	23	181
Cheese sauce packet mix, made with whole milk	6	N	N	N	N	111
Cheese sauce packet mix, made with semi-skimmed milk	3.8	N	N	N	N	91
Onion sauce, made with whole milk	6.6	2.5	1.9	1.8	10	101
Onion sauce, made with semi-skimmed milk	5.1	1.5	1.5	1.8	4	88
White sauce, savoury, made with whole milk	10.3	4	3.1	2.9	15	151
White sauce, savoury, made with semi-skimmed milk	8	2.4	2.4	2.7	6	130
Prepared and cook-in sauces						
Cook-in sauces, canned, average	0.8	0.1	0.4	0.2	tr	43
Chicken Tonight honey and mustard, Knorr	5.3	0.8	N	N	n/k	104
Chilli, Homepride	0.4	0.1	n/k	n/k	n/k	50
Green Thai, Lloyd Grossman	4.1	3.7	N	N	n/k	87
Hoi Sin, Sainsbury	tr	tr	tr	n/k	n/k	67
Indonesian satay, Sharwoods	20.5	7.8	N	N	n/k	159
Jalfrezi, Pataks	7.2	4.1	N	N	n/k	112

Food type	Total fat (g)	Sat (g)	Mono (g)	Poly (g)	Chol (mg)	Cal (kcal)
Sweet chilli, Sharwoods	0.4	tr	n/k	tr	n/k	217
Sweet and sour sauce, canned, average	0.1	0.1	0	0	0	44
Tikka Masala, Uncle Ben	6.8	N	N	N	n/k	102
Cooking sauces, sweet						
Custard, made with whole milk	4.5	2.9	1.2	0.2	16	118
Custard, made with semi-skimmed milk	2	1.2	0.5	0.1	7	95
Custard, ready to use, average	2.9	0	0.8	0.1	2	98
White sauce, sweet, made with whole milk	9.5	3.6	2.8	2.6	14	171
White sauce, sweet, made with semi-skimmed milk	7.4	2.2	2.2	2.5	6	152
Ice cream topping, average	0.2	tr	tr	tr	0	207
Condiments and gravies						
Gravy, instant granules, dry weight	32.5	N	N	N	N	462

TIP: Harissa, the North African chilli and spice paste, is now much easier to find. Strength varies across different brands so go easy to start with, but it can be invaluable. A little stirred into a plain bean soup will give it oomph, and it is delicious with roast vegetables. It is also a useful ingredient for marinades and makes a great dip when stirred into a mixture of low-fat crème fraîche and 0 per cent fat Greek yoghurt with some chopped fresh coriander.

Food type	Total fat (g)	Sat (g)	Mono (g)	Poly (g)	Chol (mg)	Cal (kcal)
Gravy, instant, made up	2.4	N	N	N	N	34
Meat extract, e.g. Bovril	0.6	N	N	N	N	179
Pepper, black	3.3	N	N	N	0	N
Pepper, white	2.1	N	N	N	0	N
Salt	0	0	0	0	0	N
Stock cubes, beef	9.2	3.5	3.3	1.4	tr	n/k
Stock cubes, chicken	15.4	N	N	N	tr	237
Stock cubes, vegetable	17.3	N	N	N	0	253
Tomato purée	0.3	tr	0.1	0.1	0	76
Vinegar	0	0	0	0	0	22
Yeast extract, e.g. Marmite	0.4	N	N	N	0	180
For more pasta sauces, see *Pasta and pizza*						
Herbs and spices are all acceptable in realistic quantities						

DAIRY

Always make heart-friendly choices when it comes to dairy products, as many are high in fats, calories and – in the case of cheese – salt. Try lower-fat products like yoghurt (but check for added sugars, which can increase calorie content), crème fraîche and fromage frais. Wean yourself off full-cream milk gradually if you find it difficult to swap to skimmed immediately, but keep that as your target, or try soya milk – comparable to semi-skimmed milk in overall fat content but lower in saturates and with the added benefits of soya. Some brands of soya milk can easily be confused with cow's milk, even in hot drinks. Processed cheeses can be particularly high in salt, as can Danish Blue and Feta, so eat them in moderation and rinse the latter in cold water before use.

TIP: Try to incorporate more soya in your diet, as it can reduce the level of LDLs ('bad cholesterol') in many people. Or choose soya milk and soya yoghurt, and experiment with ingredients like tofu – soya bean curd.

Food type	Total fat (g)	Sat (g)	Mono (g)	Poly (g)	Chol (mg)	Cal (kcal)
Milks						
Skimmed milk	0.2	0.1	0.1	tr	3	32
Skimmed milk, pasteurised	0.3	0.1	0.1	tr	4	34
Skimmed milk, pasteurised and fortified	0.1	0.1	tr	tr	2	39
Skimmed milk, sterilised	0.3	0.3	tr	tr	2	35
Skimmed milk, UHT	0.1	N	N	tr	2	27
Semi-skimmed milk	1.7	1.1	0.4	tr	6	46
Semi-skimmed milk, pasteurised	1.7	1.1	0.4	tr	6	46
Semi-skimmed milk, pasteurised and fortified	1.6	1	0.5	tr	7	51
Semi-skimmed milk, UHT	1.6	1.1	0.4	tr	7	46
Whole milk	3.9	2.5	1	0.1	14	66
Whole milk, pasteurised	3.9	2.5	1	0.1	14	66
Whole milk, sterilised	3.9	2.4	1.1	0.1	14	66
Whole milk, UHT	3.9	2.4	1.1	0.1	14	66
Channel Island milk, whole, pasteurised	5.1	3.3	1.3	0.1	16	78
Breakfast milk, pasteurised	4.7	3	1.1	0.2	16	72
Coffeemate powder	34.9	32.1	1.1	tr	2	540

TIP: Milk that comes from organic cows, reared on grass, is higher in omega-3s than that from industrially reared cows, which are kept indoors. Eggs from organic or free-range hens are also higher in nutrients.

Food type	Total fat (g)	Sat (g)	Mono (g)	Poly (g)	Chol (mg)	Cal (kcal)
Condensed milk, whole, sweetened	10.1	6.3	2.9	0.3	36	333
Condensed milk, skimmed, sweetened	0.2	0.1	0.1	tr	I	267
Dried skimmed milk, fortified	0.6	0.4	0.2	tr	12	348
Dried skimmed milk, fortified, with vegetable fat	25.9	16.8	7.3	0.7	17	487
Evaporated milk, whole	9.4	5.9	2.7	0.3	34	151
Evaporated milk, light (4% fat)	4.1	2.5	1.1	0.2	17	107
Flavoured milk, strawberry and banana	1.5	1	0.3	0.1	7	64
Flavoured milk, chocolate	1.5	1	0.4	0.1	7	63
Milkshake, thick	1.8	1.2	0.4	0.1	11	88
Goat's milk, pasteurised	3.7	2.4	1	0.2	11	62
Sheep's milk	5.8	3.6	1.5	0.3	12	93
Soya milk, sweetened, plus calcium	2.4	0.4	0.5	1.4	0	43
Soya milk, unsweetened	1.6	0.2	0.3	1.1	0	26
Soya milk, unsweetened, Alpro light	1.2	0.2	0.3	0.7	0	21

TIP: One way of cutting down on the amount of cream for use to top fresh fruit is to whisk it half-and-half with 0 per cent fat Greek yoghurt. Gradually work your way towards replacing the cream completely.

Food type	Total fat (g)	Sat (g)	Mono (g)	Poly (g)	Chol (mg)	Cal (kcal)
Cream and cream substitutes						
Cream, fresh, single	19.1	12.2	5.1	0.6	55	193
Cream, fresh, double	53.7	33.4	13.8	1.9	137	496
Cream, fresh, whipping	40.3	25.2	11.7	1.1	105	381
Cream, fresh, clotted	63.5	39.7	18.4	1.8	170	586
Cream, sour	19.9	12.5	5.8	0.6	60	205
Cream, sterilised, canned	23.9	14.9	6.9	0.7	65	239
Crème fraîche	40	27.1	8.6	1.1	113	378
Crème fraîche, half fat	15	10.2	3.2	0.4	N	162
Dairy cream, UHT, canned spray	24.2	15.2	6.1	0.8	68e	252
Dairy cream, UHT, canned spray, 'light'	17.3	10.9	4.3	0.6	46	196
Dairy cream, extra thick	23.5	15.3	6	0.8	74	236
Dream Topping, using semi-skimmed milk	11.7	10.5	0.5	0.1	6	166
Elmlea, single	14.5	9.2	3.2	1.3	4e	158
Elmlea, double	35.7	24.3	6.5	2.8	11e	345
Elmlea, whipping	29.9	26.4	2.8	0.9	8	292
'Top' dessert topping	6.5	5.9	0.2	0.1	4	112

TIP: Low-fat versions of dairy products are easily found, but don't forget about other foods that are comparatively low in fat anyway, such as ricotta and fromage frais. The latter is a good substitute for crème fraîche.

Food type	Total fat (g)	Sat (g)	Mono (g)	Poly (g)	Chol (mg)	Cal (kcal)
Cheese						
Babybel	23	N	N	N	N	299
Brie	29.1	18.2	6.7	0.6	93	343
Caerphilly	31	21.1	7.9	0.7	90	371
Camembert	22.7	14.2	6.6	0.7	72	290
Cheddar	34.9	21.7	9.4	1.1	97	416
Cheddar type, lower fat	15.8	9.9	4.6	0.4	43	273
Cheddar, vegetarian	32	20.8	8.7	1.2	105	390
Cheese spread, plain	22.8	15.8	5.8	0.8	67	267
Cheese spread, reduced fat	9.5	6.6	2.4	0.3	N	175
Cheshire	31.8	21.1	7.9	0.7	90	371
Cottage cheese, plain	4.3	2.3	1.2	0.2	16	101
Cottage cheese, plain, reduced fat	1.5	1	0.4	tr	5	79
Cottage cheese with extra ingredients, average	3.8	2.4	1.1	0.1	13	95
Cream cheese	47.4	29.7	13.7	1.4	95	439
Danish blue	28.9	19.1	7.5	1	75	342
Double Gloucester	34.5	21.6	10.1	1	100	402
Edam	26	15.8	5.2	0.4	71	341
Feta	20.2	13.7e	4.1e	0.6e	70	250

TIP: Probiotic yoghurts may seem to be good for you, but check the sugar content. Without any sweetening they would be unpalatable, and the quantity of sugar can be as much as 18 per cent.

Food type	Total fat (g)	Sat (g)	Mono (g)	Poly (g)	Chol (mg)	Cal (kcal)
Goats' milk soft cheese, full fat	25.8	17.9	6.1	1	93	320
Gouda	30.6	20.3	7.4	0.9	85	377
Lancashire	31.8	21.1	7.9	0.7	90	371
Mozzarella, fresh	20.3	13.8	5	0.8	58	257
Parmesan, fresh	29.7	19.3	7.7	1.1	93	415
Processed cheese, plain	23	14.3	6.3	0.8	85	297
Processed cheese slices, reduced fat	13.3	8.1	3.6	0.5	48e	228
Red Leicester	34.5	21.6	10.1	1	100	402
Roule, garlic and herb	27	20	N	N	N	295
Spreadable cheese, soft white, full fat	31.3	20.5	7.8	1	92	132
Spreadable cheese, soft white, medium fat	16.3	10.7e	4e	0.5e	48e	199
Spreadable cheese, soft white, low fat	8	5.2e	2e	0.3e	24e	312
Stilton, blue	35	23	9.2	1.2	95	410
Wensleydale	31.8	21.1	7.9	0.7	90	380
Yoghurts, etc.						
Whole milk, plain	3	1.7	0.9	0.2	11	79
Whole milk, fruit	3	2	0.7	0.1	3	109

TIP: Calcium doesn't just come from dairy products. Other sources include the bones of tinned fish and green leafy vegetables, as well as calcium-fortified products and tofu.

Food type	Total fat (g)	Sat (g)	Mono (g)	Poly (g)	Chol (mg)	Cal (kcal)
Children's whole milk, fruit	3.7	2.5	0.9	0.1	4	90
Twinpot, whole milk, with fruit	3.2	N	N	N	N	106
Low fat, plain	1	0.7	0.2	tr	1	56
Low fat, fruit	1.1	0.8e	0.3e	tr	0e	78
Diet, plain	0.2	0.1e	0.1e	tr	N	54
Diet, fruit	0.2	0.1e	0.1e	tr	N	47
Greek style, plain	10.2	6.8	2.5	0.3	17	133
Greek style, fruit	8.4	5.6	2.2	0.2	14	137
Greek style, lower fat	2.7	2	N	N	N	80
Greek – sheep's milk	6	4.2	1.6	0.2	14e	92
Greek – 0% fat	0	0	0	0	0e	52
Soya yoghurt, fruit	1.8	0.3	0.4	1.1	0	73
Yoghurt drinks, fortified yoghurts etc.						
Activia, Danone	0.1	tr	n/k	n/k	n/k	56
Drinking yoghurt, UHT, average	tr	tr	tr	tr	tr	62
Lassi, yoghurt drink, sweetened	0.9	0.6	0.2	tr	N	62
Strawberry drink, Actimel	1.5	1.1	n/k	n/k	n/k	74
Vanilla Drink, Müller Vitality	1.7	1	n/k	0.1	n/k	77
Yoghurt, classic strawberry, Benecol	0.6	tr	n/k	n/k	n/k	78

TIP: Make a quick smoothie by blending low-fat natural yoghurt, skimmed milk and half a ripe banana. Add a drop or two of vanilla essence if you wish.

Food type	Total fat (g)	Sat (g)	Mono (g)	Poly (g)	Chol (mg)	Cal (kcal)
Yoghurt drink, Yakult	0.1	n/k	n/k	n/k	n/k	74
Yoghurt, reduced sugar, Flora ProActiv	0.5	0.1	n/k	n/k	n/k	55
Fromage frais						
Fromage frais, plain	8	5.5	1.8	0.2	9	113
Fromage frais, fruit	5.6	3.5	1.6	0.2	20	124
Fromage frais, virtually fat free, plain	0.1	0.1	tr	tr	1	49
Fromage frais, virtually fat free, fruit	0.2	0.1	0.1	tr	1	50
For butter, see *Oils and fats*						
For smoothies, see *Drinks*						
For ice creams, see *Desserts and puddings*						

TIP: If you cook with low-fat yoghurt or other similar products they will probably separate. Add a little flour before use to stabilise them – whisk it in well.

DESSERTS AND PUDDINGS

Fresh fruit is one of the best desserts; you are getting all the nutritional benefits without any of the unhealthy ingredients that might be included in a prepared dessert or ready meal. If you are making your own puddings, experiment; many recipes work just as well if you reduce the fat and sugar content. Ice cream desserts can be among the better choices, and meringues are good – provided they are not filled with lots of high-fat whipped cream and you cut back on the sugar. Fresh fruit salad is one of the best options when entertaining or eating out, but be careful about any made with sugar syrups if you're trying to lose weight.

TIP: Stir pieces of broken meringue into Greek yoghurt very gently, and then mix in some chopped strawberries. Serve immediately.

Food type	Total fat (g)	Sat (g)	Mono (g)	Poly (g)	Chol (mg)	Cal (kcal)
Hot desserts and puddings						
Bread pudding	9.5	N	N	N	52	289
Christmas pudding, retail, average	11.8	6.1	4.1	0.6	36	329
Crumble, fruit, average	8.3	4	3.1	0.7	12	219
Crumble, fruit, wholemeal	7.4	1.5	2.3	3.2	0	195
Lemon meringue pie	8.5	3.1	3.5	1.5	12	251
Pancackes, made with whole milk	16.3	7	6.6	1.7	68	302
Milk pudding (e.g. rice), made with whole milk	4.3	2.7	1.1	0.2	15	130
Rice pudding, canned	1.3	0.8	0.3	0.1	9e	85
Rice pudding, canned, low fat	0.8	0.5e	0.2e	0.1e	N	71
Sponge pudding, average, canned	9.1	5	3	0.5	32	265
Treacle tart	14.2	4.4	5.3	3.6	7	379
Cold desserts						
Banoffee pie	20	N	N	N	N	319
Cheesecake, frozen	16.2	9.4	5	0.8	92	294

TIP: Melt a little 70 per cent chocolate in a bowl over a pan of boiling water. Brush the tops of four meringue nests with the melted chocolate and set aside until cool. Chop some fresh strawberries, pile them inside each meringue nest and top with a dollop of low-fat crème fraîche.

Food type	Total fat (g)	Sat (g)	Mono (g)	Poly (g)	Chol (mg)	Cal (kcal)
Cheesecake, fruit, individual	12.3	7.5	3.5	0.5	15	264
Chocolate dairy desserts, average	10.7	6.3	3.3	0.4	21	214
Crème caramel	1.6	0.9	0.5	0.1	N	104
Jelly, made with water	0	0	0	0	0	61
Meringue	tr	tr	tr	tr	0	381
Meringue with cream	24.2	15.1	7	0.7	63	330
Mousse, chocolate	6.5	3.3	2.7	0.1	N	149
Mousse, chocolate, reduced fat	3.7	2.5	0.9	0.1	1	123
Mousse, fruit	6.4	4.1	1.8	0.1	N	143
Pavlova, frozen, with fruit and cream	13.2	7.3	4.6	0.7	30	288
Pavlova, frozen, varieties with cream but no fruit	19.7	10.8	6.8	1	45	370
Profiteroles with sauce, frozen	25.7	14	8.7	1.7	N	345

TIP: Granitas have been described as 'slushies for adults'. For a lemon granita to serve 4, gently heat 125g caster sugar with 600ml water and the thinly pared rind of 3 organic lemons. When the sugar is dissolved, boil the mixture for 5 minutes. Add the lemon juice, allow it to cool, and strain. Pour it into a freezer container, seal and freeze for 2 hours. Whisk and return to the freezer for another 2 hours. Whisk again and freeze until firm – it's supposed to have crystals. Leave it at room temperature for about 5 minutes before serving, then stir until the crystals break up a bit.

Food type	Total fat (g)	Sat (g)	Mono (g)	Poly (g)	Chol (mg)	Cal (kcal)
Sorbet, fruit	0.3	N	N	N	0	97
Torte, fruit	15.5	9.4	4.7	1.2	42	258
Trifle, home-made, average	8.1	2.4	2.6	1.7	21	166
Trifle, retail, fruit	9	5.6	2.5	0.4	13	164
Ice creams						
Cherry Garcia frozen yoghurt, Ben & Jerry's	3	N	N	N	N	160
Choc ice	21.7	18.4	1.9	0.4	7	295
Chocolate nut sundae, home-made, average	14.9	8.6	4.3	0.9	28	243
Chocolate coated ice cream bar, average (e.g. Snickers)	23.3	12.5	7.8	1.3	N	311
Cornetto-type cones, average	17.8	13.2	3.2	0.6	15	284
Cream of Cornish, Walls	4	2.7	N	N	N	83
Dairy ice cream, vanilla	9.8	6.1	2.8	0.3	24	177

TIP: Atholl Brose is a delicious and comparatively heart-friendly dessert when you make the 'healthy' version. To serve 2 generously (or 4 less so) mix 150g zero per cent fat Greek yoghurt and the same quantity of low-fat crème fraîche. Toast 2 tablespoons of oatmeal and one of chopped almonds in a dry frying pan over a medium heat until they begin to change colour. Add them to the yoghurt and stir well. Then add a tablespoon each of whisky and heather honey and mix again. Put the mixture into serving dishes and chill for at least an hour. Serve straight from the fridge

Food type	Total fat (g)	Sat (g)	Mono (g)	Poly (g)	Chol (mg)	Cal (kcal)
Dairy ice cream, vanilla premium	15.1	9.1	4.4	0.6	N	215
Dairy Milk luxury ice cream, Cadbury	5.7	3.2	N	N	N	155
Ice cream, vanilla, non-dairy	7.8	4.8	2.2	0.4	7	153
Lollies, containing ice cream	3.8	2.1	1.2	0.3	4	118
Lollies, real fruit juice	0.3	N	N	N	N	73
Pralines and cream, Haagen Dazs	15.1	N	N	N	N	242
Spagnola, Carte d'or	5.7	N	N	N	N	188
Vanilla, Ben & Jerry's	15	N	N	N	N	225
Vienetta, vanilla, Walls	17	N	N	N	N	254
Toppings and sauces						
Custard, made with whole milk	4.5	2.9	1.2	0.2	16	118

TIP: Make a delicious apricot dessert. For 4 people, put 250g unsulphurated dried apricots in a pan and add the finely chopped zest and juice from a large, unwaxed orange (if the orange isn't very juicy,use two). Add a few drops of vanilla essence and 2 tsp of clear honey. Then bring the fruit to the boil, reduce the heat and place a lid partly over the pan. Simmer the apricots for about 20 minutes. Put them in a serving bowl with the remaining juice and leave them to cool. This dessert is rich and sweet as well as comparatively good for you. A little goes a long way.

Food type	Total fat (g)	Sat (g)	Mono (g)	Poly (g)	Chol (mg)	Cal (kcal)
Custard, made with						
semi-skimmed milk	2	1.2	0.5	0.1	7	95
Custard, ready to eat	2.9	0	0.8	0.1	2	98
Ice cream topping, average	0.2	tr	tr	tr	0	207
Ice cream wafers	0.7	N	N	N	0	342
For fruit pies, see *Pies and quiches*						

TIP: Make a fruit purée and use that as a sauce for desserts rather than cream or custard. Hot raspberry purée is particularly successful and if the fruit is very sweet, you won't need to add much sugar.

DRINKS

The main problem with alcohol isn't fat content, it's calories – and the effect it has on your willpower. Keep to sensible drinking limits and don't be tempted into drinking loads of red wine just because it can provide some protection against heart disease. Non-alcoholic fizzy drinks can also be high calorie, so check labels and watch portion sizes: most cans contain 330ml, but the nutritional information quoted on cans and bottles is often for 100ml. Both tea and coffee are best drunk black; at the very least milk should be skimmed. Watch out for powdered coffee drinks and coffeeshop coffees – see pages 233–6, as they can be particularly high in saturated fat.

TIP: Cut down on the milk you use in tea or coffee; if you don't already do so, then aim to take them both black. Black tea is better when made with quality tea, brewed for a short time and served with a slice of lemon.

Food type	Total fat (g)	Sat (g)	Mono (g)	Poly (g)	Chol (mg)	Cal (kcal)
Alcoholic drinks						
Advocaat	6.3	N	N	N	N	272
Bailey's Irish Cream	N	N	N	N	N	320
Beer, bitter	tr	tr	tr	tr	0	30
Beer, bitter, premium/best	tr	tr	tr	tr	0	33
Beer, keg	tr	tr	tr	tr	0	31
Beer, draught	tr	tr	tr	tr	0	32
Beer, mild, draught	tr	tr	tr	tr	0	25
Brandy	0	0	0	0	0	222
Brown ale, bottled	tr	tr	tr	tr	0	30
Cherry brandy	0	0	0	0	0	262
Cider, dry	0	0	0	0	0	36
Cider, sweet	0	0	0	0	0	42
Cider, vintage	0	0	0	0	0	101
Cider, low alcohol	0	0	0	0	0	17
Cognac	0	0	0	0	0	350
Cointreau	0	0	0	0	0	340
Curacao	0	0	0	0	0	311
Gin	0	0	0	0	0	222
Grand Marnier	0	0	0	0	0	320
Lager	tr	tr	tr	tr	0	29
Lager, premium	tr	tr	tr	tr	0	59
Lager, low alcohol	tr	tr	tr	tr	0	10
Lager, alcohol free	tr	tr	tr	tr	0	7
Pale ale, bottled	tr	tr	tr	tr	0	28

Food type	Total fat (g)	Sat (g)	Mono (g)	Poly (g)	Chol (mg)	Cal (kcal)
Port	0	0	0	0	0	157
Rum	0	0	0	0	0	222
Shandy, canned	0	0	0	0	0	24
Sherry, dry	0	0	0	0	0	116
Sherry, medium	0	0	0	0	0	116
Sherry, sweet	0	0	0	0	0	136
Stout	tr	tr	tr	tr	0	30
Strong ale / barley wine	tr	tr	tr	tr	0	66
Tia Maria	0	0	0	0	0	262
Vermouth, dry	0	0	0	0	0	109
Vermouth, sweet	0	0	0	0	0	151
Vodka	0	0	0	0	0	222
Whisky	0	0	0	0	0	222
Wine, red	0	0	0	0	0	68
Wine, rose	0	0	0	0	0	71
Wine, white, dry	0	0	0	0	0	66
Wine, white, medium	0	0	0	0	0	74
Wine, white, sweet	0	0	0	0	0	94
Wine, white, sparkling	0	0	0	0	0	74
Fruit juices and squashes						
Apple juice, fresh, unsweetened	0.1	tr	tr	0.1	0	38
Blackcurrant juice drink, undiluted	0	0	0	0	0	288
Cranberry juice	0	0	0	0	0	49
Fruit squash, average, undiluted	tr	tr	tr	tr	0	93

Food type	Total fat (g)	Sat (g)	Mono (g)	Poly (g)	Chol (mg)	Cal (kcal)
Fruit squash, low calorie, undiluted	tr	tr	tr	tr	0	3
Fruit juice drink, ready to drink	tr	tr	tr	tr	0	37
Fruit juice drink, ready to drink, low calorie	tr	tr	tr	tr	0	10
Grape juice, unsweetened	0.1	tr	tr	tr	0	46
Grapefruit juice, unsweetened	0.1	tr	tr	tr	0	33
Lemon juice, fresh	tr	tr	tr	tr	0	7
Lime juice cordial, undiluted	0	0	0	0	0	112
Orange juice, unsweetened	0.1	0.1	tr	tr	0	36
Pineapple juice, unsweetened	0.1	tr	tr	tr	0	41
Sunny Delight	0.2	tr	tr	tr	tr	39
Tomato juice	tr	tr	tr	tr	0	14
Smoothies						
Apple and blackcurrant, Sainsbury	tr	tr	n/k	n/k	0	64
Blackberries and blueberries, PJs	tr	tr	n/k	n/k	0	56
Kids' orange, mango and pineapple, Innocent	0.1	tr	n/k	n/k	0	44
Mango and passion-fruit, Innocent	0.3	0.1	n/k	n/k	0	56
Strawberry and banana, Innocent	0.1	tr	n/k	n/k	0	55
Fizzy drinks						
Bitter lemon	tr	tr	tr	tr	0	35

Food type	Total fat (g)	Sat (g)	Mono (g)	Poly (g)	Chol (mg)	Cal (kcal)
Cola	0	0	0	0	0	41
Cola, diet	0	0	0	0	0	1
Elderflower pressé	0	0	0	0	0	35
Fruit drinks, averaged	tr	tr	tr	tr	0	39
Ginger ale, dry	0	0	0	0	0	15
Ginger beer	0	0	0	0	0	35
Lemonade	0	0	0	0	0	22
Lucozade	0	0	0	0	0	60
Tonic water	0	0	0	0	0	33
Other drinks, including powdered						
Bournvita powder	1.5	N	N	N	N	341
Build-up powder, shake	1.1	0.6	0	0	12e	347
Cocoa powder	21.7	12.8	7.2	0.6	0	312
Coffees						
Coffee, infusion, average	tr	tr	tr	tr	0	2
Coffee, instant	tr	tr	tr	tr	0	75
Coffee and chicory essence	0.2	tr	tr	tr	0	218
Cappuccino mix, unsweetened, Nestlé	23.8	23.9	n/k	n/k	n/k	464
Cappuccino mix, standard, Nestlé	17.4	17.2	n/k	n/k	n/k	444
Cappuccino mix, low fat, Nestlé	4.8	4.7	n/k	n/k	n/k	365
Latte mix, Nestlé	28.5	28.2	n/k	n/k	n/k	498
Latte mix, caramel, Nestlé	14.1	14	n/k	n/k	n/k	423

Food type	Total fat (g)	Sat (g)	Mono (g)	Poly (g)	Chol (mg)	Cal (kcal)
Latte mix, Irish cream, Nestlé	14.1	14	n/k	n/k	n/k	425
Latte mix, vanilla, Nestlé	14.9	14.8	n/k	n/k	n/k	429
Mocha mix, Nestlé	13.1	13	n/k	n/k	n/k	418
Mocha mix, double chocolate, Nestlé	11	10.9	n/k	n/k	n/k	408
Complan powder, original and sweet varieties	14.8	6.6	6.3	1.6	N	441
Complan powder, savoury	14.6	6.2	5.9	1.6	N	432
Drinking chocolate powder	5.8	3.4	1.8	0.3	0	373
Drinking chocolate, made with whole milk	4	2.6	1.1	0.2	13	90
Drinking chocolate, made with semi-skimmed milk	2	1.3	0.5	0.1	5	73
Drinking chocolate powder, reduced fat	2.3	1.3e	0.7e	0.1e	tr	354
Horlicks powder	4.7	N	N	N	N	373
Instant drink powder, chocolate, low calorie	11.1	8.1	1.7	0.9	3	359
Instant drink powder, malted	9.5	8.7	0.2	0.1	5	416
Milk shake powder, average	1.6	N	N	N	tr	388
Ovaltine powder	1.9	1	N	N	N	352
Tea	tr	tr	tr	tr	0	tr
For coffee shop drinks, see *Fast food and takeaways*						

EGGS

Eggs can safely be eaten in moderation unless you have been specifically told to avoid them. Though egg yolks are very high in cholesterol, current studies suggest that saturated fat is the element in the diet that affects blood cholesterol levels the most. No research has yet shown that people who eat a lot of eggs are more prone to heart attacks than people who eat very few. Cook them without fat and enjoy them – they are low in saturated fat, high in protein, folic acid and other B vitamins. Opt for organic eggs if you can as there is some evidence that these have the highest levels of nutrients.

TIP: Egg whites have no cholesterol, virtually no saturated fats – or other fats – so make the most of meringues. Just be careful about what you have with them. Substitute low-fat crème fraîche for cream, for example.

Food type	Total fat (g)	Sat (g)	Mono (g)	Poly (g)	Chol (mg)	Cal (kcal)
Eggs						
Chicken eggs, raw weight	11.2	3.2	4.4	1.7	391	151
White of egg, raw	tr	tr	tr	tr	0	36
Yolk, raw	30.5	8.7	13.2	3.4	1120	339
Boiled	10.8	3.1	4.7	1.2	385	147
Fried in vegetable oil	13.9	4	6	1.5	435	179
Poached	10.8	3.1	4.7	1.2	385	147
Duck eggs, raw weight	11.8	2.9	4.9	2	680	163
Egg dishes						
Omelette, plain	16.8	7.2	5.6	1.7	357	195
Omelette, cheese	23	12.2	6.9	1.5	268	271
Scrambled eggs, made with milk and butter	23.4	11.6	7.3	1.9	361	257

TIP: Don't go mad and try to cut out all fats. Research has shown that very low-fat diets might actually be bad for people who are either at risk of developing coronary heart disease or who already have it.

FISH AND SEAFOOD

Increasing the amount of fish, particularly oily fish, you eat is one of the most beneficial changes you can make to your diet. Try to eat at least two portions of fish a week, with at least one being oily fish – mackerel, salmon, tuna, herring, trout: darker-fleshed fish, essentially. Many varieties of shellfish (and squid) contain high levels of cholesterol, but this is thought to have little direct effect on blood cholesterol. If you already enjoy these there's no need to stop eating them, but don't go mad either – you should be fine unless your doctor has specifically advised you to avoid them. They are useful sources of vitamin B12 and several other nutrients.

TIP: Make marinated kippers. For 4 people, skin 8 fillets and put in a shallow china or glass dish (don't use metal) with a finely sliced onion, 8 peppercorns and a bay leaf. Spoon over a couple of tablespoons of olive oil, and one of cider vinegar. Cover the dish and leave to marinate for 24 hours, during which time you turn the fillets a couple of times. They don't need cooking; just drain them and serve with wholemeal bread.

Food type	Total fat (g)	Sat (g)	Mono (g)	Poly (g)	Chol (mg)	Cal (kcal)
White fish						
Cod fillet, raw weight	0.7	0.1	0.1	0.3	46	80
Cod, baked with butter	1.2	0.3e	0.2e	0.4e	56e	96
Cod, poached in milk with butter	1.1	0.3e	0.1e	0.3e	53e	94
Cod, frozen steaks, raw weight	0.6	0.1	0.1	0.2	39	72
Cod, frozen steaks, grilled	1.3	0.4	0.2	0.3	49e	95
Cod in batter, fried in blended oil	15.4	1.6	5.5	7.5	N	247
Cod in crumbs, fried in blended oil or oven baked	14.3	1.5e	5.2e	7e	N	235
Cod in parsley sauce, boiled	2.8	N	N	N	N	84
Cod, dried and salted, boiled	0.9	0.2	0.1	0.4	59	138
Coley, raw weight	1	0.1	0.3	0.3	40e	82
Coley, steamed	1.3	0.2	0.3	0.4	55	105
Haddock fillet, raw weight	0.6	0.1	0.1	0.2	36	81
Haddock fillet, steamed	0.6	0.1	0.1	0.2	38	89
Haddock in crumbs, fried in blended oil or oven baked	10	N	N	N	N	196
Haddock, smoked, steamed	0.9	0.2e	0.1e	0.3e	47e	101
Halibut, grilled	2.2	0.4	0.7	0.5	41	121
Lemon sole, raw weight	1.5	0.2	0.3	0.5	60	83
Lemon sole, steamed	0.9	0.1	0.2	0.3	73	91
Lemon sole goujons, baked	14.6	N	N	N	N	187
Lemon sole goujons, fried in blended oil	28.7	2.9e	11.4e	12.3e	53	374

Food type	Total fat (g)	Sat (g)	Mono (g)	Poly (g)	Chol (mg)	Cal (kcal)
Monkfish, fillet, raw weight	0.4	0.1	0.1	0.1	N	70
Plaice, raw weight	1.4	0.2	0.4	0.3	42	79
Plaice, frozen, steamed	1.5	0.2	0.4	0.4	54	92
Plaice in batter, fried in blended oil	16.8	1.8	6.1	8.2	N	257
Plaice in breadcrumbs, fried in blended oil	13.7	1.5	4.9	6.7	N	228
Plaice goujons, baked	18.3	N	N	N	N	304
Plaice goujons, fried in blended oil	32.3	3.4e	12.9e	13.3e	22	426
Rock salmon (dogfish), in batter, fried in blended oil	21.9	2.9e	8e	9.9e	N	295
Skate in batter, fried in blended oil	10.1	1	3.4	4.7	N	168
Whiting, steamed	0.9	0.1	0.3	0.2	55	92
Whiting in crumbs, fried in blended oil	10.3	1.1	3.7	5	N	191
Oily fish						
Anchovies, canned in oil, drained	10	1.6	5.3	1.8	63	191
Eel, jellied	7.1	1.9	3.5	1	79	98

TIP: Try barbecuing fresh sardines, a great source of omega-3s: buy them cleaned, brush with olive oil and cook over hot charcoal until they're lightly charred. Serve with lemon wedges.

Food type	Total fat (g)	Sat (g)	Mono (g)	Poly (g)	Chol (mg)	Cal (kcal)
Herring, raw weight	13.2	3.3	5.5	2.7	50	190
Herring, grilled	11.2	2.8	4.7	2.3	43	181
Kipper, raw weight	17.7	2.8	9.3	3.9	64	229
Kipper, grilled	19.4	3.1	10.2	4.2	70	255
Mackerel, raw weight	16.1	3.3	7.9	3.3	54	220
Mackerel, grilled	17.3	3.5	8.5	3.5	58	239
Mackerel, smoked	30.9	6.3e	15.1e	6.3e	105	354
Pilchards, canned in tomato sauce	8.1	1.7	2.2	3.4	56	144
Salmon, raw weight	11	1.9	4.4	3.1	50	180
Salmon steaks, grilled	13.1	2.5	5.8	4.1	60	215
Salmon steaks, steamed	11.9	2	4.7	3.3	54	194
Salmon, smoked	4.5	0.8e	1.8e	1.3e	35	142
Salmon, smoked, premium Shetland, Tesco	9.9	2.6	3.4	3.9	N	180
Salmon, pink, canned in brine and drained	6.6	1.3	2.4	1.9	28	153
Sardines, canned in brine, drained	9.6	N	N	N	60	172
Sardines, canned in oil, drained	14.1	2.9	4.8	5	65	220

TIP: Fish oils seem to have the effect of lowering blood triglycerides – another reason to include oily fish in your diet once or twice a week.

Food type	Total fat (g)	Sat (g)	Mono (g)	Poly (g)	Chol (mg)	Cal (kcal)
Sardines, canned in tomato sauce	9.9	2.8	2.9	3.2	76	162
Trout, rainbow, grilled	5.4	1.1	2	1.7	70	135
Tuna, canned in brine, drained	0.6	0.2	0.1	0.2	51	99
Tuna, canned in oil, drained	9	1.5	2.3	4.8	50	189
Whitebait, in flour, fried	47.5	N	N	N	N	525
Seafood						
Cockles, boiled	0.6	0.2	0.1	0.2	53	53
Crab, fresh, boiled	5.5	0.7	1.5	1.6	72	128
Crab, white meat, canned in brine	0.5	0.1e	0.1e	0.1e	72e	77
Lobster, boiled	1.6	0.2	0.3	0.6	110	103
Mussels, boiled	2.7	0.5	0.4	1	58	104
Prawns, boiled	0.9	0.2	0.2	0.2	280e	99
Prawns, tiger, whole (weighed with shells)	0.4	0.1	0.2	0.1	105	80
Scampi in breadcrumbs, fried in blended oil	13.6	1.4	5.1	6.4	110	237
Shrimps, frozen	0.8	0.1e	0.2e	0.3e	130e	73
Shrimps, canned in brine	1.2	0.2	0.3	0.4	130e	94
Squid, frozen, raw	1.5	0.3	0.2	0.5	200	70
Squid in batter, fried in blended oil	10	2.1	3.3	3.7	145	195
Whelks, boiled	1.2	0.2	0.2	0.3	125	89
Winkles, boiled	1.2	0.2	0.2	0.4	105	72

Food type	Total fat (g)	Sat (g)	Mono (g)	Poly (g)	Chol (mg)	Cal (kcal)
Fish dishes and products						
Cod roe, hard, coated and fried in blended oil	11.9	1.6	4.1	5.7	315	202
Crabsticks	0.4	N	N	N	39e	68
Fish balls, Chinese, steamed	0.5	N	N	N	N	74
Fish cakes, fried in blended oil	13.4	1.8	5.4	5.6	21	218
Fish curry, Bangladeshi	8	N	N	N	N	127
Fish fingers, cod, fried in blended oil	14.1	3.6e	5.3e	4.6e	32	238
Fish fingers, cod, grilled	8.9	2.8	3.4	2.3	35	200
Fish paste, average	10.5	N	N	N	N	170
Fisherman's pie, retail, average	5.4	1.8	1.3	0.7	N	118
Prawn curry	8.5	1.4	3.8	2.9	144	117
Prawns with vegetables, Chinese	4.7	0.7	2.4	1.4	56	83
Salmon en croute, retail	19.1	3.1	2.9	1.4	31	288
Seafood cocktail	1.5	0.3	0.2	0.5	115e	87
Seafood pasta, retail	4.8	2.8	1.2	0.3	41	110
Smoked haddock kedgeree, made with rice and egg	9.1	2.1e	3e	3.1e	126e	176
Taramasalata	52.9	4.1	29.3	16.7	25	504
Tuna pâté	18.6	7.8	4.4	5.3	72	236

FRUIT

People who include lots of fruit and vegetables in their diet have fewer heart attacks than people who don't. Remember the guideline of five portions a day. Like vegetables, fruits are high in antioxidants and contain many other valuable nutrients. Always eat the skin of fruits like apples and pears (washing them first) as they are a good source of fibre. With such a variety of fruits available, everybody can find something they like. Make a point of having at least one piece of fresh fruit every day, in place of a less healthy snack, and choose fresh fruit for desserts.

TIP: Bananas cooked in the dying embers of a barbecue make a delicious low-fat dessert. Bake them, in their skins, in the charcoal for about 20–30 minutes; the skins will turn black. Remove them once they are soft, peel and sprinkle with brown sugar. They are also delicious drizzled with a little rum!

Food type	Total fat (g)	Sat (g)	Mono (g)	Poly (g)	Chol (mg)	Cal (kcal)
Apples, cooking, raw weight	0.1	tr	tr	0.1	0	35
Apples, puréed with sugar	0.1	tr	tr	0.1	0	74
Apples, puréed with no sugar	0.1	tr	tr	0.1	0	33
Apples, eating, raw	0.1	tr	tr	0.1	0	47
Apples, eating, peeled	0.1	tr	tr	0.1	0	45
Apricots, raw	0.1	tr	tr	tr	0	31
Apricots, semi-dried, 'ready to eat'	0.6	N	N	N	0	158
Apricots, canned in juice	0.1	tr	tr	tr	0	34
Apricots, canned in syrup	0.1	tr	tr	tr	0	63
Avocado, average	19.5	4.1	12.1	2.2	0	190
Bananas	0.3	0.1	tr	0.1	0	95
Blackberries	0.2	tr	0.1	0.1	0	25
Blackberries, stewed with sugar	0.2	tr	0.1	0.1	0	56
Blackcurrants, raw	tr	tr	tr	tr	0	28
Blackcurrants, stewed with sugar	tr	tr	tr	tr	0	58
Blueberries, fresh	0.2	0	tr	tr	0	30
Blueberries, dried	1	0.2	0.2	0.5	0	330
Cherries, raw	0.1	tr	tr	tr	0	48
Cherries, canned in syrup	tr	tr	tr	tr	0	71
Cherries, glacé	tr	tr	tr	tr	0	251
Cherry pie filling	tr	tr	tr	tr	0	82
Clementines	0.1	tr	tr	tr	0	37
Cranberries, dried	0.8	tr	0.4	0.3	0	360

Food type	Total fat (g)	Sat (g)	Mono (g)	Poly (g)	Chol (mg)	Cal (kcal)
Currants	0.4	N	N	N	0	267
Damsons, raw	tr	tr	tr	tr	0	38
Damsons, stewed with sugar	tr	tr	tr	tr	0	74
Dates, raw	0.1	tr	tr	tr	0	124
Dates, dried	0.2	tr	tr	tr	0	270
Dried mixed fruit	0.4	N	N	N	0	268
Figs, dried	1.6	N	N	N	0	227
Figs, ready to eat	1.5	N	N	N	0	209
Fruit cocktail, canned in juice	tr	tr	tr	tr	0	29
Fruit cocktail, canned in syrup	tr	tr	tr	tr	0	57
Fruit pie filling	tr	N	N	N	0	77
Fruit salad, home-made	0.1	tr	tr	tr	0	60
Gooseberries, raw weight	0.4	N	N	N	0	19
Gooseberries, stewed with sugar	0.3	N	N	N	0	54
Grapefruit, raw	0.1	tr	tr	tr	0	30
Grapefruit, canned in juice	tr	tr	tr	tr	0	30
Grapefruit, canned in syrup	tr	tr	tr	tr	0	60
Grapes, black and white, average	0.1	tr	tr	tr	0	60

TIP: Use organic citrus fruit if you can, as pesticides can penetrate the skins. You get more juice from a warm lemon, too, so if you keep them in the fridge take them out a couple of hours before you want to use them.

Food type	Total fat (g)	Sat (g)	Mono (g)	Poly (g)	Chol (mg)	Cal (kcal)
Guava, raw	0.5	N	N	N	0	26
Guava, canned in syrup	tr	tr	tr	tr	0	60
Kiwi fruit	0.5	N	N	N	0	49
Lemon	0.3	0.1	tr	0.1	0	19
Lychees, raw	0.1	tr	tr	tr	0	58
Lychees, canned in syrup	tr	tr	tr	tr	0	68
Mandarin oranges, canned in juice	tr	tr	tr	tr	0	32
Mandarin oranges, canned in syrup	tr	tr	tr	tr	0	52
Mango, raw	0.2	0.1	tr	tr	0	57
Mango, dried	1	0.6	0.1	0.3	0	350
Melon, cantaloupe	0.1	tr	tr	tr	0	19
Melon, galia	0.1	tr	tr	tr	0	24
Melon, honeydew	0.1	tr	tr	tr	0	28
Mixed peel	0.9	N	N	N	0	231
Nectarines	0.1	tr	tr	tr	0	40
Oranges	0.1	tr	tr	tr	0	37
Passion-fruit	0.4	0.1	0.1	0.1	0	36
Paw-paw, raw	0.1	tr	tr	tr	0	36

TIP: Melons are a good choice for a heart-friendly diet, and a plate spread with slices of different varieties looks appetising. A melon is ripe when the flesh gives slightly at the stem end, and chilling a whole melon in the fridge for about an hour will give a clear, fresh taste.

Food type	Total fat (g)	Sat (g)	Mono (g)	Poly (g)	Chol (mg)	Cal (kcal)
Paw-paw, canned in juice	tr	tr	tr	tr	0	65
Peaches, raw	0.1	tr	tr	tr	0	33
Peaches, canned in juice	tr	tr	tr	tr	0	39
Peaches, canned in syrup	tr	tr	tr	tr	0	55
Pears, raw	0.1	tr	tr	tr	0	40
Pears, canned in juice	tr	tr	tr	tr	0	33
Pears, canned in syrup	tr	tr	tr	tr	0	50
Pineapple, raw	0.2	tr	0.1	0.1	0	41
Pineapple, canned in juice	tr	tr	tr	tr	0	47
Pineapple, canned in syrup	tr	tr	tr	tr	0	64
Plums, average, raw	0.1	tr	tr	tr	0	36
Plums, stewed with sugar	0.1	tr	tr	tr	0	79
Plums, canned in syrup	tr	tr	tr	tr	0	59
Prunes, canned in juice	0.2	tr	0.1	0.1	0	79
Prunes, canned in syrup	0.2	tr	0.1	0.1	0	90
Prunes, ready to eat	0.4	N	N	N	0	141
Raisins	0.4	N	N	N	0	272
Raspberries, raw	0.3	0.1	0.1	0.1	0	25
Raspberries, canned in syrup	0.1	tr	tr	tr	0	88

TIP: Berries, especially blueberries, can be useful in combating cholesterol. Blueberries contain a lot of the antioxidant anthocyanin, a pigment that gives them their deep colour, and a small serving of half a cupful has as many antioxidants as five servings of broccoli, peas, apples or carrots.

Food type	Total fat (g)	Sat (g)	Mono (g)	Poly (g)	Chol (mg)	Cal (kcal)
Rhubarb, raw weight	0.1	tr	tr	tr	0	7
Rhubarb, stewed with sugar	0.1	tr	tr	tr	0	48
Rhubarb, canned in syrup	tr	tr	tr	tr	0	31
Satsumas	0.1	tr	tr	tr	0	36
Strawberries, raw	0.1	tr	tr	tr	0	27
Strawberries, canned in syrup	tr	tr	tr	tr	0	65
Sultanas	0.4	tr	tr	tr	0	275
Tangerines	0.1	tr	tr	tr	0	35
Watermelon	0.3	0.1	0.1	0.1	0	31
Olives						
Olives in brine, green	11	1.7	5.7	1.3	0	103
Olives in brine, black	16.9	2.3	11.9	1	0	155
Olives, green , pepper-stuffed, Tesco	12.6	2.4	9	0.7	0	135
Olives, mixed, with lemon and garlic, Cypressa	18.9	2.9	N	N	0	176

TIP: Frozen seedless black grapes can be an impressive end to a dinner party, and are refreshing on a hot day. Wash sprigs of grapes, about 10–12 grapes each, and freeze. Use them straight from the freezer, allowing them to rest for a couple of minutes before eating.

JAMS, MARMALADES AND SPREADS

Most sweet spreads contain a high proportion of sugar, and the same is often true of savoury chutneys. Though their fat content may be comparatively low, calories can be very high, so monitor quantities carefully and make wise choices when shopping – for example, investigating fruit spreads rather than jams. Nut butters can be very high in fat and it is important to be selective. Some peanut butters, for example, contain palm oil – and palm oil has twice as much saturated fat as peanut oil. Spreads like Marmite may appear to be high in salt, but the average portion is small – about half a teaspoonful (2.5g). Marmite is also high in vital B vitamins.

TIP: Using food products that contain plant sterols and are advertised as reducing cholesterol may be helpful for people who are already at risk – but they are not a substitute for modifying an unhealthy diet.

Food type	Total fat (g)	Sat (g)	Mono (g)	Poly (g)	Chol (mg)	Cal (kcal)
Sweet spreads						
Chocolate spread	37.6	N	N	N	2	569
Fruit purée spread	0.1	tr	tr	tr	0	121
Honey	0	0	0	0	0	288
Jam						
Black cherry, Tiptree	tr	0	0	0	0	268
Damson, Sainsbury	0.1	tr	n/k	n/k	0	264
Fruit with edible seeds, average	0	0	0	0	0	261
Reduced sugar, average	0.1	tr	tr	tr	0	123
Raspberry, Robertson	0.1	0.1	0	0	0	243
Rhubarb and ginger, Tiptree	tr	n/k	n/k	n/k	0	268
Stone fruit, e.g. apricot, average	0	0	0	0	0	261
Lemon curd, average	4.9	1.5	2	1.2	21	282
Marmalade	0	0	0	0	0	261
Nut butters						
Almond butter	56.1	4.7	N	N	0	633
Chocolate and hazelnut spread, average, e.g. Nutella	33	10.1	16.8	4.6	2	549
Peanut butter, smooth	51.8	12.8	19.9	16.8	0	606
Peanut butter, crunchy, organic	48.2	8.6	N	N	0	606
Tahini paste (sesame seed)	58.9	8.4	22	25.8	0	634
Tahini paste, dark	58.4	9.9	N	N	0	678
Savoury spreads						
Meat extract, e.g. Bovril	0.6	N	N	N	N	179
Yeast extract, e.g. Marmite	0.4	N	N	N	0	180

MEAT AND POULTRY

Cutting back on meat, particularly on red meat, can be one of the most significant heart-friendly changes you can make. Reduce portion sizes – don't have more than three thin slices or a piece bigger than the size of a deck of cards. Remove visible fat, and the skin from poultry, and you also reduce the quantity of saturated fat substantially. Try to cut out meat-based ready meals; by avoiding them you not only control the amount and type of fat in your food, but you also avoid a lot of extra salt.

TIP: Marinate meat for kebabs for 1–3 hours before assembling and barbecuing or grilling. Lemon juice, olive oil and chopped shallots make a good marinade for both chicken and lamb, and you don't need much. Use a shallow bowl and turn the cubes of meat regularly, or put the meat and the marinade into a resealable plastic bag. Seal, shake well, and put in the fridge. You'll need to shake it several times before cooking.

Food type	Total fat (g)	Sat (g)	Mono (g)	Poly (g)	Chol (mg)	Cal (kcal)
Bacon and ham						
Bacon rashers, back, raw weight	16.5	6.2	6.9	2.2	53	215
Bacon rashers, back, fat trimmed, raw weight	6.7	2.5	2.8	0.9	31e	136
Bacon rashers, back, dry-fried	22	8.3	9.2	2.8	65	295
Bacon rashers, back, grilled	21.6	8.1	9	2.8	75	287
Bacon rashers, back, fat trimmed, grilled	12.3	4.6	5.2	1.6	44	214
Bacon rashers, back, grilled crispy	18.8	7.1	7.9	2.4	68	313
Bacon rashers, back, microwaved	23.3	8.8	9.8	3	84	307
Bacon rashers, back, reduced salt, grilled	20.6	7.8	8.7	2.7	74	282
Bacon rashers, middle, grilled	23.1	8.4	10	3	83	307
Bacon rashers, streaky, raw weight	23.6	8.2	10.2	3.5	65	276
Bacon rashers, streaky, grilled	26.9	9.8	11.5	3.7	90	337
Bacon rashers, streaky, fried	26.6	9.1	11.1	4.5	78	335
Gammon joint, raw weight	7.5	2.5	3.3	1.2	23	138
Gammon, boiled	12.3	4.1	5.4	1.9	83	204
Gammon rashers, grilled	9.9	3.4	4.1	1.7	83	199
Ham, cooked, average	3.3	1.1	1.4	0.5	58	107
Beef						
Beef, trimmed lean, raw weight	4.3	1.7	1.9	0.2	58	129

Food type	Total fat (g)	Sat (g)	Mono (g)	Poly (g)	Chol (mg)	Cal (kcal)
Braising steak, cooked, lean	9.7	4.1	4.1	0.6	100	225
Braising steak, cooked, lean and fat	12.7	5.3	5.2	0.8	100	246
Fore rib or rib roast, raw weight	19.8	8.9	8.8	0.7	59	253
Fore rib or rib roast, cooked	20.4	9.2	9.1	0.7	83	300
Mince, raw weight, average	16.2	6.9	6.9	0.5	60	225
Mince, microwaved	17.5	7.6	7.7	0.7	80	263
Mince, cooked	13.5	5.7	5.7	0.6	79	209
Mince, extra lean, cooked	8.7	3.8	3.8	0.3	75	177
Rump steak, raw weight, lean and fat	10.1	4.3	4.4	0.6	60	174
Rump steak, barbecued, lean	5.7	2.4	2.4	0.4	76	176
Rump steak, fried, lean	6.6	2.4	2.5	0.9	86	183
Rump steak, fried, lean and fat	12.7	4.9	5.2	1.6	84	228
Rump steak, grilled, lean	5.9	2.5	2.5	0.5	76	177
Rump steak strips, stir-fried, lean	8.8	3.3	3.5	1.2	92	208
Rump steak, steakhouse, lean	4.7	2	2	0.3	73	162

TIP: Roast meat without adding any extra fat. Cover the top with foil, if necessary, and stand the joint on a rack in the roasting tin so the fat runs out. If you normally roast potatoes by putting them under the joint then do them in another dish, and cook them with olive or rapeseed oil. Remember that you are trying to avoid saturated fats.

Food type	Total fat (g)	Sat (g)	Mono (g)	Poly (g)	Chol (mg)	Cal (kcal)
Silverside, salted, boiled, lean	6.9	2.5	3.4	0.3	74	184
Stewing steak, raw weight, lean and fat	6.4	2.6	2.9	0.4	69	146
Stewing steak, cooked, lean and fat	9.6	3.7	4.2	0.9	91	203
Topside, raw weight, lean and fat	12.9	5.4	5.8	0.8	48	198
Topside, roasted, well done, lean meat	6.3	2.6	2.8	0.3	88	202
Topside, roasted, well done, lean and fat	12.5	5.2	5.7	0.6	83	244
Lamb						
Lamb, average, trimmed, raw weight	8	3.5	3.1	0.5	74	153
Best end neck cutlets, raw weight, lean and fat	27.9	13.6	10.4	1.4	76	316
Best end neck cutlets, grilled, lean	13.8	6.5	5.1	0.7	100	238
Best end neck cutlets, grilled, lean and fat	29.9	14.5	11.2	1.5	105	367
Breast, roasted, lean	18.5	8.6	7	0.9	95	273
Breast, roasted, lean and fat	29.9	14.3	11.4	1.4	93	359
Leg, average, raw weight, lean and fat	12.3	5.4	4.9	0.7	78	187
Leg, roasted medium, lean	9.4	3.8	3.9	0.6	100	203

Food type	Total fat (g)	Sat (g)	Mono (g)	Poly (g)	Chol (mg)	Cal (kcal)
Leg, roasted medium, lean and fat	14.2	5.7	6.1	0.8	100	305
Loin chops, raw weight, lean and fat	23	10.8	8.8	1.2	79	277
Loin chops, grilled, lean	10.7	4.9	4	0.6	96	213
Loin chops, grilled, lean and fat	22.1	10.5	8.4	1.3	100	305
Loin chops, microwaved, lean and fat	26.9	12.8	10.2	1.5	110	352
Loin chops, roasted, lean and fat	26.9	12.8	10.2	1.5	113	359
Mince, average, raw weight	13.3	6.2	5.3	0.6	77	196
Mince, cooked	12.3	5.8	4.8	0.6	96	208
Neck fillet strips, stir-fried, lean	20	8.2	7.6	2.2	86	278
Shoulder, raw weight, lean and fat	18.3	8.5	7.1	1	76	235
Shoulder, diced, grilled	19.3	9	7.5	1	110	288
Shoulder, roasted, lean	12.1	5.5	4.7	0.6	105	218
Shoulder, roasted, lean and fat	22.1	10.4	8.7	1	105	298
Stewing lamb, pressure cooked, lean	14.8	6.5	5.6	1	100	248
Stewing lamb, stewed, lean	14.8	6.5	5.6	1	94	240
Stewing lamb, stewed, lean and fat	20.1	9.2	7.7	1.3	92	279
Pork						
Pork, average, trimmed lean, raw weight	4	1.4	1.5	0.7	63	123

Food type	Total fat (g)	Sat (g)	Mono (g)	Poly (g)	Chol (mg)	Cal (kcal)
Pork, trimmed fat, raw weight	56.4	20.4	23.7	9.5	71	548
Pork fat, cooked (crackling)	50.9	17.9	21.5	8.9	98	515
Belly pork, grilled, lean and fat	23.4	8.2	9.5	4	97	320
Diced pork, casseroled, lean only	6.4	1.9	2.3	1.6	99	184
Fillet strips, stir-fried, lean	5.9	1.3	1.8	2.2	90	182
Leg joint, raw weight, lean and fat	15.2	5.1	6.4	2.5	63	213
Leg joint, roasted medium, lean	5.5	1.9	2.3	0.7	100	182
Leg joint, roasted medium, lean and fat	10.2	3.6	4.4	1.4	100	215
Loin chops, raw weight, lean and fat	21.7	8	8.5	3.6	61	270
Loin chops, barbecued, lean and fat	15.8	5.7	6.3	2.6	87	255
Loin chops, grilled, lean	6.4	2.2	2.6	1	75	184
Loin chops, grilled, lean and fat	15.7	5.6	6.5	2.5	86	257
Loin chops, microwaved, lean and fat	14.1	4.9	5.7	2.5	100	248
Loin chops, roasted, lean and fat	19.3	7	7.8	3.1	110	301
Steaks, raw weight, lean and fat	9.4	3.3	3.8	1.6	63	169
Steaks, grilled, lean and fat	7.6	2.7	3	1.2	100	198

TIP: Skinning raw chicken breasts is easy. Grip one edge of the skin and pull it back and away from the meat, lifting it off. If necessary, remove any remaining pieces with a knife.

Food type	Total fat (g)	Sat (g)	Mono (g)	Poly (g)	Chol (mg)	Cal (kcal)
Veal						
Veal escalope, raw weight	1.7	0.6	0.7	0.3	52	106
Veal escalope, fried	6.8	1.8	2.5	1.9	110	196
Rabbit						
Rabbit, raw weight, meat only	5.5	2.1	1.3	1.8	53	137
Stewed, meat only	3.2	1.7	0.7	0.6	49	114
Venison						
Venison, roasted	2.5	N	N	N	N	165
Offal						
Heart, lamb, roasted	13.9	N	N	N	260	226
Kidney, lamb, fried	10.3	N	N	N	610	188
Kidney, ox, stewed	4.4	1.4	1	0.9	460	138
Kidney, pig, stewed	6.1	2	1.6	0.9	700	153
Liver, calf, fried	9.6	N	N	N	330	176
Liver, chicken, fried	8.9	N	N	N	350	169
Liver, lamb, fried	12.9	N	N	N	400	237
Liver, ox, coated in flour and stewed	9.5	3.5	1.5	2	240	198
Liver, pig, coated in flour and stewed	8.1	2.5	1.3	2.2	290	189
Oxtail, stewed	13.4	N	N	N	110	243
Tongue, sheep, cooked	24	N	N	N	270e	289
Tripe, dressed, raw weight	0.5	0.2	0.2	tr	64	33
Trotters and tails, boiled	22.3	N	N	N	N	280

Food type	Total fat (g)	Sat (g)	Mono (g)	Poly (g)	Chol (mg)	Cal (kcal)
POULTRY						
Chicken						
Dark meat, raw weight	2.8	0.8	1.3	0.6	105	109
Light meat, raw weight	1.1	0.3	0.5	0.2	70	106
Meat, average, raw weight	2.1	0.6	1	0.4	90	108
Breast, casseroled, meat only	5.2	1.5	2.4	1	90	160
Breast, grilled without skin, meat only	2.2	0.6	1	0.4	94	148
Breast strips, stir-fried	4.6	N	N	N	87	161
Breast in crumbs, fried	12.7	2.1	5.3	4.6	33e	242
Drumsticks, roasted, meat and skin	9.1	2.5	4.3	1.8	135	185
Roasted, meat, average	7.5	2.9	5.1	2.2	120	177
Roasted, dark meat	10.9	1	1.6	0.7	82	196
Roasted, light meat	0.8	1.4	1.7	1.1	100	153
Roasted leg quarter, meat and skin	16.9	4.6	7.8	3.2	115	236
Roasted wing quarter, meat and skin	14.1	3.9	6.4	2.7	100	226
Skin, crisply roasted/grilled	46.1	12.9	22.5	7.7	170	501
Turkey						
Dark meat, raw weight	2.5	0.8	1	0.6	86	104

TIP: Cut down on the amount of meat used in casseroles; substitute pulses instead. Haricot or borlotti beans are especially good.

Food type	Total fat (g)	Sat (g)	Mono (g)	Poly (g)	Chol (mg)	Cal (kcal)
Light meat, raw weight	0.8	0.3	0.3	0.2	57	105
Meat, average, raw weight	1.6	0.5	0.6	0.4	70	105
Breast, fillet, grilled, meat only	1.7	0.6	0.6	0.3	74	155
Breast strips, stir-fried	4.5	N	N	N	72	164
Roasted, meat, average	4.6	1.4	1.7	1.1	100	166
Roasted, dark meat	6.6	2	2.4	1.7	120	177
Roasted, light meat	2	0.7	0.7	0.5	82	153
Skin, crisply roasted/grilled	40.2	13.2	15.6	8.8	290	481
Duck						
Duck, raw weight, meat only	6.5	2	3.2	1	110	137
Roasted, meat only	10.4	3.3	5.2	1.3	115	195
Roasted, meat, fat and skin	38.1	11.4	19.3	5.3	99	423
Crispy, Chinese style	24.2	7.2e	12.3e	3.4e	63e	331
Goose, roasted – meat, fat and skin	21.2	6.6e	9.9e	2.4e	91e	301
Pheasant, roasted, meat only	12	4.1	5.6	1.6	220e	220
Meat and poultry products						
Beefburgers, chilled or frozen, raw weight	24.7	10.7	11.4	0.5	76	291
Beefburgers, fried	23.9	10.7	10.8	0.8	96	329
Beefburgers, grilled	24.4	10.9	11.2	0.7	75e	326
Economy burgers, frozen, raw weight	21.2	8	9.4	2.1	92e	261
Economy burgers, grilled	19.3	7.3	8.6	1.9	84	273

Food type	Total fat (g)	Sat (g)	Mono (g)	Poly (g)	Chol (mg)	Cal (kcal)
Grill steaks, chilled or frozen, grilled	23.9	10.8	10.7	0.8	88	305
Black pudding	21.5	8.5e	8.1e	3.6e	68	297
Chicken nuggets	13	3.3	6.8	2.2	55	265
Chicken pie, individual	17.7	7	7.4	2.4	32	288
Chicken roll	4.8	1.5	2.1	0.9	40	131
Chicken wings, marinated, chilled or frozen	16.6	4.6	7.5	3.3	120e	274
Corned beef	10.9	5.7	4.3	0.3	84	205
Cornish pasty	16.3	5.9	8.4	1.2	33	267
Frankfurter	25.4	9.2	11.5	3	76	287
Game pie	22.5	7.9	9	4	60	381
Haggis, boiled	21.7	7.6	6.9	1.4	91	310
Liver sausage	16.7	5.3	5.7	2.3	115	226
Luncheon meat, canned	23.8	8.7	11	3	64	279
Meat-based pie, average	26.7	8.4	7.8	1.9	39	310
Meat spread, average beef and ham	13.4	5.5	5.8	1.2	62	192
Parma ham, Asda	16.1	5.8	8.5	1.1	n/k	224
Pâté, liver	32.7	9.5	11.8	3	170	348
Pâté, meat, reduced fat	12	3.5	3.9	1.5	160	191
Pâté de campagne, Tesco	22	8	9.9	3.1	n/k	266
Pâté, farmhouse with mushroom, Tesco	34.5	13	15	6.2	n/k	367
Polony	21.2	N	N	N	40	281

Food type	Total fat (g)	Sat (g)	Mono (g)	Poly (g)	Chol (mg)	Cal (kcal)
Pork pie	25.7	9.7	11	3.2	45	363
Salami, average	39.2	14.6	17.7	4.4	83	438
Salami, Danish	47.5	17.7	21	6.7	60	454
Salami, German	25	10.3	11.3	2.9	n/k	309
Salami, Milano	33.1	11.2	15.9	5.9	n/k	406
Sausages, beef, grilled	19.5	7.9	8.8	1.4	42	278
Sausages, pork, raw weight	25	9.2	11.2	3.4	60	309
Sausages, pork, fried	23.9	8.5	10.3	3.5	53	308
Sausages, pork, grilled	22.1	8	9.6	3	53	294
Sausages, reduced fat, grilled	13.8	4.9	5.9	2.1	55	230
Sausages, premium, grilled	22.4	8.2	9.4	3.3	72	292
Sausage rolls	27.6	11.2	N	N	N	383
Saveloy	22.3	7.5	9.8	3.6	78	296
Scotch eggs	16	4.3	6.8	2.8	165	241
Stewed steak with gravy, canned	10.1	4.7	4.4	0.3	38	158
Tongue slices	14	6	6.4	0.9	115	201
Turkey roll	9	2.7	3.8	2	150	166
White pudding	31.8	N	N	N	22	450
Related cooking ingredients						
Gelatine	0	0	0	0	0	338
Suet, shredded	86.7	49.9	30.4	2.2	82	826
Meat dishes						
Beef bourguignon	6.3	2.1	2.9	0.9	42	122

Food type	Total fat (g)	Sat (g)	Mono (g)	Poly (g)	Chol (mg)	Cal (kcal)
Beef bourguignon, made with lean beef	4.3	1.3	2	0.7	40	105
Beef casserole, using cook-in sauce	6.5	2.7	2.9	0.4	44	136
Beef chow mein	6	1.3	3.1	1.4	N	136
Beef curry, chilled or frozen, reheated	6.6	3.1	2.5	0.6	32	137
Beef curry with rice	3.9	1.8	1.4	0.3	18	131
Beef goulash	3	0.9	1.4	0.5	17	79
Beef stew	4.6	1.5	2.1	0.6	35	107
Beef stir-fried with green peppers	8	2.7	3.7	1.1	32	141
Chicken curry, chilled/frozen, with rice	5	2.2	1.6	0.8	28	145
Chicken curry, made with canned chicken sauce	6.5	N	N	N	72	150
Chicken in white sauce, canned	8.3	2.3	3.9	1.6	49	141
Chicken tandoori, chilled	10.8	3.3	5	2	120	214
Chicken, stir-fried with rice and vegetables, frozen	4.6	N	N	N	N	132

TIP: Portion size is the key and we're all accustomed to larger portions than we were in the past. Check yours, especially of higher fat foods like meat, and cut them back. A serving the size of the back of your clenched fist is about right for chicken.

Food type	Total fat (g)	Sat (g)	Mono (g)	Poly (g)	Chol (mg)	Cal (kcal)
Chilli con carne, chilled or frozen, with rice	2.7	1.1	1.1	0.1	N	107
Coq au vin	11	4.2	4.4	1.6	67	155
Coronation chicken	31.7	5.3	8.5	15.9	89	364
Cottage or shepherd's pie, chilled or frozen	5.4	2.4	2.2	0.4	16	111
Faggots in gravy, chilled / frozen	7.5	2.5	2.9	1	45	148
Irish stew, made with standard lamb	6.2	2.9	2.3	0.4	27	118
Irish stew, made with lean lamb	4.9	2.2	1.8	0.3	26	107
Irish stew, canned	5.1	2.5	2	0.3	15	91
Lamb curry, made with canned curry sauce	18.9	N	N	N	63	249
Lamb/beef hotpot, chilled/frozen	4.4	1.7	1.9	0.5	N	108
Moussaka, chilled/frozen	8.3	2.9	3.6	1.1	26	140
Pork casserole, made with cook-in sauce	7.8	2.7	3.2	1.4	50	154
Spaghetti Bolognese, chilled or frozen, sauce only	5.7	2.3	2.5	0.5	N	108
Steak and kidney pie, home-made	15.1	4.9	5.8	3.5	112	261
Accompaniments						
Dumplings	11.7	6.6	4	0.5	11	208
Stuffing mix, dried	5.2	2.4	1.6	0.1	5	338

Food type	Total fat (g)	Sat (g)	Mono (g)	Poly (g)	Chol (mg)	Cal (kcal)
Stuffing, sage and onion, home-made (using egg)	15.1	3.1	4.7	5.9	54	269
Yorkshire pudding	10.1	5.2	3.5	0.6	69	210

TIP: Small amounts of trans fats are found naturally in meat and dairy products, but they are mainly created artificially during hydrogenation, a process that converts liquid vegetable oil into solid fat. They are used in the commercial manufacture of food – so check labels on biscuits, ready meals, sausages and even chocolate snacks – and are linked with increased rates of heart disease.

NUTS AND SEEDS

There has been some research indicating that nuts can have a beneficial effect on blood lipids, which could be because most of the fat they contain is unsaturated. This is good news, so try and incorporate a few nuts into your diet every day – scatter chopped walnuts over a spinach salad or stir toasted almonds into low-fat Greek yoghurt. The benefits of nuts are not shared by coconut, however, which is high in saturates. Seeds are a great source of essential fatty acids and protein, and also have high levels of vitamins and minerals. Remember that nuts are high in calories, though, and be sparing with the quantity you use.

TIP: Toasting almonds is easy. Spread split ones on a baking sheet and pop under the grill for a few minutes until they begin to brown; keep an eye on them as they can catch quickly.

Food type	Total fat (g)	Sat (g)	Mono (g)	Poly (g)	Chol (mg)	Cal (kcal)
Nuts						
Almonds	55.8	4.4	38.2	10.5	0	612
Almonds, ground	56	5	N	N	0	632
Brazil nuts	68.2	16.4	25.8	23	0	682
Cashew nuts, roasted	50.9	10.1	29.4	9.1	0	611
Chestnuts	2.7	0.5	1	1.1	0	170
Hazelnuts	63.5	4.7	50	5.9	0	650
Macadamia nuts	77.6	11.2	60.8	1.6	0	748
Mixed nuts (peanuts, almonds, cashews, hazelnuts)	54.1	8.4	28.2	14.8	0	607
Peanut and raisin mix	25.9	4.9	12.3	7.3	0	435
Peanuts, plain	46	8.7	22	13.1	0	563
Peanuts, dry roasted	49.8	8.9	22.8	15.5	0	589
Peanuts, roasted	53	9.5	24.2	16.5	0	602
Pecan nuts	70.1	5.7	42.5	18.7	0	689
Pine nuts	68.6	4.6	19.9	41.1	0	688
Pistachio nuts, roasted	55.4	7.4	27.6	17.9	0	601
Trail mix	28.5	N	N	N	0	432
Walnuts	68.5	5.6	12.4	47.5	0	688

TIP: Toasted pumpkin and sunflower seeds make a great garnish for salads or soups, or add crunch to something like a baked potato. They are simple to toast in a dry frying pan over a medium heat; keep stirring them about and remove the pan from the heat once they begin to colour. Allow them to cool.

Food type	Total fat (g)	Sat (g)	Mono (g)	Poly (g)	Chol (mg)	Cal (kcal)
Nut products						
Almond butter	56.1	4.7	N	N	0	633
Marzipan, home-made, using egg	25.8	2.2	17.4	4.8	29	462
Marzipan, white and yellow, retail	12.7	1	8	3.1	0	389
Peanut butter, crunchy, organic	48.2	8.6	N	N	0	606
Peanut butter, smooth	51.8	12.8	19.9	16.8	0	606
Coconut and coconut products						
Coconut, dessicated	62	53.4	3.5	1.5	0	604
Coconut, creamed, block	68.8	59.3	3.9	1.6	0	669
Coconut milk, fresh	0.3	0.2	tr	tr	0	22
Coconut milk, canned, low fat	9.8	9.4	n/k	n/k	0	105
Seeds and seed products						
Linseeds/flaxseeds	34	0	N	N	0	460
Pumpkin seeds	45.6	8	11.2	18.3	0	569
Sesame seeds	58	8.3	21.7	25.5	0	598

TIP: Buy whole nuts in relatively small quantities and keep them in a cool place, and they should be fine for 2–3 months. Shelled nuts deteriorate more quickly, going rancid, and should be used promptly. It's worth investing in a good nutcracker – they often appear in the shops around Christmas and then vanish until the following year.

Food type	Total fat (g)	Sat (g)	Mono (g)	Poly (g)	Chol (mg)	Cal (kcal)
Sunflower seeds	47.5	4.5	9.8	31	0	581
Tahini paste, light, average (sesame seed)	58.9	8.4	22	25.8	0	634
Tahini paste, dark, average	58.4	9.9	N	N	0	678

TIP: Don't forget about the need to reduce salt levels, and ensure that you don't make things worse by eating salted nuts. If you find peanuts unappetising without salt, try hazelnuts or almonds instead.

OILS AND FATS

The type of fat or oil you use is vital in a cardio-protective diet, as explained on pages 37–47. When saturated fat is replaced in the diet by monounsaturated fat, blood cholesterol levels seem to be lowered. Go for olive oil – virgin, extra virgin or just ordinary – or rapeseed oil when you need a neutral taste. When choosing spreads, check out the nutritional panels carefully, maintaining healthy scepticism about health claims. Avoid any with 'hydrogenated' or 'partly hydrogenated' fats, which are trans fats by another name. Remember that sterol-enriched spreads are only of benefit if they form part of a healthy diet; they're not an alternative to it.

TIP: Use an oil and water spray to cut down on the quantity of oil you use. Use a small, new, clean spray bottle with a mixture of one part oil to seven parts water; use either olive or rapeseed oil. Shake well before use and spray cooking surfaces, like pans, or the food itself, especially if you're going to grill it.

Food type	Total fat (g)	Sat (g)	Mono (g)	Poly (g)	Chol (mg)	Cal (kcal)
Oils						
Coconut oil	99.9	86.5	6	1.5	0	899
Corn oil	99.9	14.4	29.9	51.3	0	899
Groundnut (peanut) oil	99.9	20	44.4	31	0	899
Olive oil, including virgin and extra virgin	99.9	14.3	73	8.2	0	899
Palm oil	99.9	47.8	37.1	10.4	0	899
Rapeseed oil	99.9	6.6	59.3	29.3	0	899
Safflower oil	99.9	9.7	12	74	0	899
Sesame oil	99.7	14.6	37.5	43.4	0	899
Soya oil	99.9	15.6	21.3	58.8	0	899
Sunflower oil	99.9	12	20.5	63.3	0	899
Vegetable oil, blended – average (proportion depends on blend)	99.9	11.7	53.2	29.8	0	899
Walnut oil	99.9	9.1	16.5	69.9	0	899
Wheatgerm oil	99.9	18.6	16.6	60.4	0	899
Butter and spreads						
Butter	82.2	52.1	20.9	2.8	213	744
Butter, spreadable	82.5	45.4	22.7	3.5	280	745
Blended spread, 70–80% fat, e.g. Clover	74.8	25.5	37.5	8.5	67	680

TIP: A small pat of butter contains about the same number of calories as a teaspoon of oil – about 45 – but the oil, especially olive or rapeseed oil, is better for your heart.

Food type	Total fat (g)	Sat (g)	Mono (g)	Poly (g)	Chol (mg)	Cal (kcal)
Blended spread, 40% fat, e.g. Clover Extra Light	40.3	18.1	13.4	7.3	46	390
Dairy spread, 40% fat	40	26.8	10	1.2	N	388
Margarine, hard – e.g. Echo	79.3	34.6	36.2	5.4	285	718
Margarine, hard, vegetable fat	82.3	40	21	21.3	15	742
Margarine, soft, not polyunsaturated	81.7	27.2	38.9	12.4	275	740
Margarine, soft, polyunsaturated	82.8	17	26.6	36	2	746
Fat spread, 70–80% fat, not polyunsaturated	71.2	30.4	31.2	6.5	86	642
Fat spread, 70% fat, polyunsaturated, e.g. Vitalite	68.5	16.2	15.2	33.6	tr	622
Fat spread, 60% fat, polyunsaturated, e.g. Vitalite Light	60.8	11.3	18.1	28.6	3	553
Fat spread, 60% fat, with olive oil, e.g. Bertolli	62.7	11.3	36.4	12.5	0	569
Fat spread, 40% fat, not polyunsaturated, e.g. Gold	37.5	8.4	21	6.2	6	368

TIP: Rapeseed oil is as good for you as olive oil and has a more neutral taste, more appropriate for cooking some dishes. Check the ingredients of ordinary vegetable oils, and you may find that they are 100 per cent rapeseed oil.

Food type	Total fat (g)	Sat (g)	Mono (g)	Poly (g)	Chol (mg)	Cal (kcal)
Fat spread, 35–40% fat, polyunsaturated, e.g. Flora Extra Light	37.6	8.9	9.4	18	tr	365
Fat spread, 20–25% fat, not polyunsaturated, e.g. Outline	25.5	6.8	14	3.4	8	262
Fat spread, polyunsaturated, low fat own brands	20	3.7	7.2	9.1	tr	183
Cooking fats						
Basic cooking fat, e.g. Cookeen	99.9	49.5	41.2	5.3	425	899
Beef dripping	99	50.6	38	2.4	94	891
Ghee, butter	99.8	66	24.1	3.4	280	898
Ghee, vegetable	99.4	48.4	37	9.7	0	895
Lard	99	40.3	43.4	10	93	891
Suet, shredded	86.7	49.9	30.4	2.2	82	826
Suet, vegetable	87.9	45	26.3	12.8	0	836

TIP: You must have some fat in your diet. Vitamins A, D, E and K are fat-soluble so cannot be absorbed without fat, and you also require essential fatty acids – which the body cannot manufacture. Make sure you consume the right fat, however.

PASTA AND PIZZA

One of the problems with pasta, especially when eating out, is the frequent use of sauces that are high in fat. Opt for tomato- or vegetable-based sauces and don't choose any containing a lot of cream. Try wholemeal pasta, which is particularly good with strongly flavoured sauces, and accompany it with a green salad. It is worth making your own sauces rather than buying bottled ones; if you opt for the latter, then choose the tomato-based sauces again. Check out calorie counts, though, as some that are low in fat are still high in calories. Many pizzas can be high in both fat and calories. Make sensible choices and avoid the high-fat options with lots of cheese, pepperoni or other meats.

TIP: When cooking pasta use a large pan and plenty of boiling water. Add the pasta to the boiling water, stir it – to prevent sticking – until it reboils and then cook it quickly; don't cover the pan. Using a big pan enables the pasta to move around during cooking.

Food type	Total fat (g)	Sat (g)	Mono (g)	Poly (g)	Chol (mg)	Cal (kcal)
Pasta						
Macaroni, raw weight	1.8	0.3	0.1	0.8	0	348
Macaroni, boiled	0.5	0.1	tr	0.2	0	86
Plain pasta, fresh, raw weight	2.4	N	N	N	N	274
Plain pasta, fresh, cooked	1.5	0.3	0.3	0.4	N	159
Plain pasta, fresh, stuffed with cheese and veg, cooked	4.6	N	N	N	N	169
Plain pasta, dry weight, durum wheat	2	0.4	n/k	n/k	0	345
Ravioli, canned in tomato sauce	2.2	0.8	0.8	0.3	6	70
Spaghetti, white, raw weight	1.8	0.2	0.2	0.8	0	342
Spaghetti, white, boiled	0.7	0.1	0.1	0.3	0	104
Spaghetti, wholemeal, raw weight	2.5	0.4	0.3	1.1	0	324
Spaghetti, wholemeal, boiled	0.9	0.1	0.1	0.4	0	113
Spaghetti, canned in tomato sauce	0.4	0.1	0.1	0.2	0	64
Wholewheat fusilli, dry weight, Tesco	2.5	0.5	n/k	n/k	0	325
Wholewheat penne, dry weight, Tesco	1.8	0.4	n/k	n/k	0	330
Pasta dishes						
Macaroni cheese, average	9.9	4.9	2.8	1.6	21	162
Seafood pasta, retail	4.8	2.8	1.2	0.3	41	110
Lasagne, home-made, average	10.8	4.5	3.8	1.4	26	191

Food type	Total fat (g)	Sat (g)	Mono (g)	Poly (g)	Chol (mg)	Cal (kcal)
Lasagne, chilled / frozen, 10–20% meat	6.1	2.8	2.2	0.7	18	143
Pasta with meat and tomato sauce, average	3.6	1.4	1.3	0.4	11	101
Spaghetti Bolognese, chilled or frozen	2.9	1.1	1.2	0.4	N	106
Ready-made pasta sauces						
Pasta sauce, tomato based, average	1.5	0.2	0.3	0.8	0	47
Arrabbiata sauce, Sainsbury Be Good to Yourself	3.9	0.6	2.5	0.6	n/k	71
Basilico sauce, Buitoni	5.8	0.7	N	N	n/k	92
Bolognese sauce, Dolmio	1.2	1	tr	tr	n/k	53
Bolognese sauce, light, Dolmio	0.1	0	tr	tr	n/k	37
Carbonara sauce, Asda	16.5	10.3	5	0.9	n/k	148
Four-cheese sauce, Asda	10.7	6.6	3	0.4	n/k	135
Puttanesca sauce, Sainsbury	9.7	1.5	n/k	n/k	n/k	122
Siciliana, Buitoni	4.2	0.5	N	N	n/k	70
Spicy tomato sauce, microwave, Buitoni	3.5	0.4	N	N	n/k	57
Taste of Tuscany, Dolmio	3.0	N	N	N	n/k	67
Toscana sauce, Buitoni	6.9	0.8	N	N	n/k	95
Pesto, classic, Sacla	44.3	6.5	N	N	n/k	438
Pesto, sun-dried tomato, Sacla	27.9	3.9	N	N	n/k	289

Food type	Total fat (g)	Sat (g)	Mono (g)	Poly (g)	Chol (mg)	Cal (kcal)
Pizza						
Pizza base, raw weight	4.8	N	N	N	N	290
Cheese and tomato, deep pan	7.5	3.1	2.4	1.3	13	249
Cheese and tomato, thin base	10.3	4.8	3.1	1.3	22	277
Cheese and tomato, French bread	7.8	N	N	N	N	230
Cheese and tomato, frozen	8.8	3.1	2.8	1.4	N	238
Chicken topped, chilled, average	8.3	N	N	N	N	246
Fish-based topping, average	7.5	3.2	2.5	1.3	25	226
Ham and pineapple, chilled	8.6	N	N	N	N	260
Meat-based topping, average	10.3	4	3.7	1.5	19	255
Vegetarian	6.9	N	N	N	N	216
For more pizzas, see *Fast food and takeaways*						

Tip: Using wholemeal pasta is a relatively painless way of increasing the amount of fibre in your diet. Brands differ, so hunt around for one that you like before dismissing them all as too stodgy; they have changed a lot in recent years.

PIES AND QUICHES

Either eat pastry in moderation or avoid it completely – it is generally half fat by weight, and often that fat is high in saturates. Bear in mind, too, that the fillings of pies, tarts, quiches and small pastries (whether sweet or savoury) may also be higher in fat than you might wish. Make sensible choices – broccoli quiche, or smoked salmon, rather than one with a lot of fatty bacon – and don't add high-fat accompaniments like mayo or cream. It is always a good idea to leave some of the pastry crust to one side.

TIP: Sausage rolls can be tempting, but don't give in. Not only is the pastry high in saturated fat and calories, but so is the filling.

Food type	Total fat (g)	Sat (g)	Mono (g)	Poly (g)	Chol (mg)	Cal (kcal)
Cheese and onion pastry rolls	20	9	7.1	2.2	26	327
Chicken-based pie, individual	17.7	7	7.4	2.4	32	288
Cornish pasty	16.3	5.9	8.4	1.2	33	267
Quiche, cheese and egg	22.3	9.9	7.4	3.2	133	315
Quiche, cheese and egg, wholemeal	22.5	10	7.4	3.3	133	309
Quiche Lorraine	25.5	10.6	9	4	116	358
Sausage rolls	27.6	11.2	N	N	N	383
Vegetable flan, made without eggs	14.5	5.4	6.4	3.2	15	226
Vegetable pasty	16.5	5.1	6.2	4.3	8	289
Fruit pie, one crust, average	8.2	2.5	3	2.1	4	190
Fruit pie, pastry top and bottom	13.6	4.2	5.1	3.5	7	262
Fruit pie, individual	14	5.4	6	1.8	0	356
Fruit pie, blackcurrant, pastry top and bottom	13.5	4.2	5.1	3.5	7	263
Fruit pie, wholemeal, one crust	8.3	2.5	3.1	2.2	4	185
Fruit pie, wholemeal, pastry top and bottom	13.8	4.2	5.1	3.6	7	253
Treacle tart	14.2	4.4	5.3	3.6	7	379

TIP: Remember to check the nutritional information boxes on ready meals and processed foods and don't rely on slogans on the front like 'low fat'. There are only loose regulations covering what these actually mean, so ignore them.

RICE AND NOODLES

Rice can be an important element in a heart-friendly diet, but again consider the type. Brown rice, containing more fibre and nutrients, is better for you all round, and brown basmati rice can be particularly delicious. It will, however, take longer to cook. Steer clear of fried rice and rice dishes with other high-fat ingredients, such as cream. The same is true of noodles: they can be useful and tasty, but fried ones are not so good. Noodle-based snacks and flavoured noodles are often high in additives, including salt, and shouldn't form part of a heart-friendly diet.

TIP: Brown rice has a lot more flavour than white rice, as well as being better for you. Don't expect it to be as soft as white rice even when cooked, however; it will still be a bit chewy, with a nutty taste. Soaking it for up to an hour first can reduce the cooking time.

Food type	Total fat (g)	Sat (g)	Mono (g)	Poly (g)	Chol (mg)	Cal (kcal)
Basmati rice	1.4	0.2	n/k	n/k	0	356
Brown rice, raw weight	2.8	0.7	0.7	1	0	357
Brown rice, boiled	1.1	0.3	0.3	0.4	0	141
Egg-fried rice, takeaway	4.9	0.6	2.3	1.3	19	186
Pilau rice, plain, with ghee	4.6	2.6	1.1	0.5	10	142
Risotto rice, arborio	0.4	0.2	0.1	0.1	0	350
Risotto rice, carnaroli	1.4	0.6	n/k	n/k	0	355
Savoury rice, meat and vegetable, boiled	3.5	1.1	1.3	0.6	tr	142
White rice, raw weight	0.5	N	N	N	0	359
White rice, easy cook, raw weight	3.6	0.9	0.9	1.3	0	383
White rice, easy cook, boiled	1.3	0.3	0.3	0.5	0	138
White rice, cooked and fried in vegetable oil	4.1	0.6	1.9	1.3	0	144
Rice cakes	3.6	N	N	N	N	372
Egg noodles, raw weight	8.2	2.3	3.5	0.9	30	391
Egg noodles, boiled	0.5	0.1	0.2	0.1	6	62
Pot noodles, average, made up with water	3.1	N	N	N	O	103
Rice noodles, broad, dry weight	0	0	0	0	0	371
Rice thread noodles, dry weight	1	0.3	n/k	n/k	0	382
'Straight to wok' noodles, thick	1.1	n/k	n/k	n/k	0	139
'Straight to wok' noodles, medium	1.5	n/k	n/k	n/k	0	162

SNACKS, NIBBLES AND DIPS

Many snack foods are amazingly high in fat, and in the wrong kind of fat, too. They're also frequently high calorie and high in salt, and so have no real place in a cardio-protective diet, despite the recent changes in the oils used for cooking them, changes which are becoming more widespread. Go for nibbling olives (rinsed, if in brine) or a few unsalted nuts instead of crisps or tortilla chips, and watch quantities of nuts as they are high in calories. Shop-bought dips can also be high in both fat and calories, so it is worth making your own.

TIP: For a quick dip, stir some wholegrain mustard into a pot of zero per cent fat Greek yoghurt, add a tablespoon of low-fat mayo, and some chopped fresh mint if you wish. Mix well and serve with raw vegetables.

Food type	Total fat (g)	Sat (g)	Mono (g)	Poly (g)	Chol (mg)	Cal (kcal)
Savoury snacks						
Bombay mix	32.9	4	16.2	11.3	0	503
Breadsticks	8.4	5.9	1.3	0.9	0	392
Cheese balls, Asda and Tesco	31	3.6	18.5	8.1	n/k	510
Corn snacks, average, e.g. Wotsits	31.9	11.8	12.9	5.8	0	519
Mini poppadoms	35	16	N	N	0	515
Pork scratchings	46	N	N	N	N	606
Potato chips	33.2	14.7	14.3	3.6	0	535
Potato crisps:						
Ready salted and flavoured crisps, average	34.2	14	13.7	5	0	530
Lower-fat crisps, average	21.5	9.3	8.7	2.5	0	458
Low in saturates, plain crisps	34	2.6	27	2.9	0	530
Low in saturates, cheese and onion crisps	33	2.6	25.8	2.7	0	524
Low in saturates, salt and vinegar crisps	33	2.6	26.1	2.8	0	524
Low in saturates, smoky bacon crisps	33	2.6	25.8	2.7	0	524
Asda, full-fat, ready salted crisps	32.7	3.9	7.5	20.6	tr	526
Asda, full-fat, salt and vinegar crisps	31.1	3.7	7.2	19.5	tr	514
Asda, full-fat, cheese and onion crisps	31.1	3.7	7.1	19.5	tr	517

Food type	Total fat (g)	Sat (g)	Mono (g)	Poly (g)	Chol (mg)	Cal (kcal)
Kettle chips, lightly salted	25.8	2.9	N	N	n/k	482
Kettle chips, sea salt and balsamic vinegar	25	2.6	N	N	n/k	476
Kettle chips, sea salt and black pepper	24.3	2.7	N	N	n/k	471
Potato rings, average, plain and flavoured, e.g. Hula Hoops	32	13.9	12.7	4	0	523
Pot savouries – noodles, rice, etc. – average, dry weight	10.9	N	N	N	0	365
Pot savouries, average, made up with water	3.1	N	N	N	O	103
Pringles original	36	10	N	N	0	540
Pringles sour cream and onion	35	10	N	N	0	531
Sainsbury Be Good To Yourself Rosemary & Sea Salt Pitta Chips	1.4	0.3	0.3	0.8	n/k	363
Tortilla chips	22.6	4	10.6	6.7	0	459
Tortilla chips, cool, Asda and Tesco	23	11	9	2.7	0	474
Twiglets	11.7	4.9	4.4	1.8	0	383
Olives						
Olives in brine, green	11	1.7	5.7	1.3	0	103
Olives in brine, black	16.9	2.3	11.9	1	0	155
Olives, green , pepper-stuffed, Tesco	12.6	2.4	9	0.7	0	135

Food type	Total fat (g)	Sat (g)	Mono (g)	Poly (g)	Chol (mg)	Cal (kcal)
Olives, mixed, with lemon and garlic, Cypressa	18.9	2.9	N	N	0	176
Sweet snacks						
Cereal chewy bar, average	16.4	5	8.7	1.8	N	419
Cereal crunchy bar, average	22.2	4.5	11.3	5.4	tr	468
Peanut and raisin mix	25.9	4.9	12.3	7.3	0	435
Popcorn, plain	42.8	4.3	14.5	19.7	0	593
Popcorn, sweet	20	2	6.8	9.2	18	480
Trail mix	28.5	N	N	N	0	432
Dips						
Guacamole, Tesco, full fat	21	8	10.1	1.7	n/k	210
Hummus, Tesco	26.8	2.8	14.2	8.5	0	315
Hummus, 'healthy living', Tesco	11.1	1.3	5.1	4.5	0	184
Hummus, olive and sun-dried tomato, Tesco	25	2.7	13.1	8.2	0	280
Onion and garlic, Tesco, with mayo and sour cream	48.5	6.5	27.1	12.7	n/k	460
Sour-cream based dips, average	37	N	N	N	60	360
Taramasalata, average	52.9	4.1	29.3	16.7	25	504
Tomato salsa, Tesco	1.6	0.3	0.3	9	0	49
Tsatsiki, average	4.9	2.8	1.4	0.3	N	66

SOUP

Soup can be an excellent part of any diet but pay close attention to nutritional labels and ingredient lists, even on those 'fresh and healthy' packaged soups from chiller cabinets. Again it is best to make your own, without adding lots of salt – many powdered or canned varieties can be quite high in salt, and some are sweetened as well. When preparing soup it is important to read the labels on ingredients like stock cubes (which are high in salt) and avoid using a lot of fat to start the vegetables cooking (which really isn't necessary). Don't add fried bread croutons or grated cheese as a garnish – go for a healthier alternative.

TIP: Home-made soups can be made to look extra special with garnishes – and it doesn't have to be a swirl of cream. If that's what you fancy, substitute low-fat yoghurt (but let the soup cool down a bit first). Chopped fresh herbs, diced tomatoes and finely chopped spring onions all work well, too, as does a sprig of flat-leaf parsley.

Food type	Total fat (g)	Sat (g)	Mono (g)	Poly (g)	Chol (mg)	Cal (kcal)
Fresh soup						
Broad bean and bacon, fresh, Sainsbury	2	1	0.7	0.2	n/k	49
Carrot and coriander, fresh, Covent Garden	1.3	0.8	N	N	n/k	40
Chicken, fresh, Covent Garden	5.4	2.4	N	N	N	85
Minestrone, fresh, Sainsbury	0.2	tr	0.1	0.1	n/k	31
Roasted Vegetable, fresh, Duchy Originals	2.6	0.9	N	N	n/k	43
Canned soup						
Celery, condensed, made up	3.6	0.3	N	N	n/k	47

Tip: Soups keep you feeling full for longer and can be very good for you, but try making your own so that you control the ingredients. For a stunning soup for two, rinse and chop 300g spinach. Chop a medium onion, a celery stick, several cloves of garlic and 150g potatoes. Put the wet spinach in a pan over a gentle heat and let it cook down. Put half a teaspoon of olive oil in another pan and cook the onion, celery and garlic gently; don't let them brown and add the chopped spuds after a few minutes. Then add 500 ml of water and cook until the potatoes begin to soften. Add the spinach and cook until the potatoes really are soft but don't let the spinach overcook, as that will ruin its bright green colour. Then blend, adding more liquid if necessary. Add a little salt, black pepper and nutmeg, reheat and serve.

Food type	Total fat (g)	Sat (g)	Mono (g)	Poly (g)	Chol (mg)	Cal (kcal)
Chicken, cream of	3.8	0.6	2	1	97	58
Chicken, condensed	5.8	0.8	3	1.4	4	85
Chicken, condensed, made up	2.9	0.4	1.5	0.7	2	43
Clam chowder, Spinnaker	7	2	N	N	N	90
Minestrone, canned, Heinz	0.5	0.3	0.1	0.1	1	31
Mushroom, cream of	3	0.5	1.6	0.9	1	46
Oxtail	1.7	0.6	0.6	0.2	7	44
Oxtail, canned, Heinz	0.5	0.2	N	N	n/k	39
Pea and ham, canned, Baxter's	0.5	0.1	N	N	n/k	50
Tomato, cream of	3	0.5	1.6	0.8	1	52
Tomato, condensed	6.8	1	2.6	3	1	123
Tomato, condensed, made up	3.4	0.5	1.3	1.5	tr	62
Vegetable	0.6	N	N	N	N	48
Packet soup						
Chicken noodle, made up	0.3	N	N	N	N	19
Minestrone, made up	0.4	N	N	N	0	22
Tomato, made up	1.3	0.6	0.3	tr	tr	36

TIP: Soups thicken as they cool down, especially if they contain beans or lentils. Don't be tempted into adding extra liquid when you reheat them, or that will make your hot soup much thinner than you intended.

Food type	Total fat (g)	Sat (g)	Mono (g)	Poly (g)	Chol (mg)	Cal (kcal)
Vegetable	0.3	N	N	N	0	22
Build-up powder, soup, average	8.2	3.8	tr	tr	0	377

TIP: Accompany soup with some chunks of good wholemeal bread for a satisfying meal. Wholegrains really are worth it. One large US study showed that women who ate 2.7 servings of wholegrain food a day reduced their risk of heart disease by 30 per cent. Try to move away from white, refined grains completely.

SUGAR AND SWEETENERS

Sugar may contain no fat, but it is very high in calories. For that reason alone it is worth reducing the amount you use, especially if you are trying to lose weight like many people with raised cholesterol levels. If you find it hard, try reducing gradually; it's probably better to get rid of your actual desire for sugar than substitute sweeteners. Remember that many other foods are naturally sweet, but have nutritional benefits that sugar has not: fruit, for instance, contains not only useful quantities of fibre but also antioxidants, vitamins and minerals.

TIP: You can reduce sugar gradually. First add less (eventually none) to hot drinks and breakfast cereals, then cut back on soft drinks and confectionery, then on items like biscuits. Pretty soon you'll find that the food you once loved will be too sickly for you.

Food type	Total fat (g)	Sat (g)	Mono (g)	Poly (g)	Chol (mg)	Cal (kcal)
Amber sugar crystals	0	0	0	0	0	398
Date syrup	0.1	n/k	n/k	n/k	0	292
Fructose	0	0	0	0	0	400
Glucose liquid	0	0	0	0	0	318
Golden syrup	0	0	0	0	0	298
Honey	0	0	0	0	0	288
Icing sugar	0	0	0	0	0	398
Jaggery	0	0	0	0	0	367
Malt extract	tr	tr	0	0	0	294
Maple syrup	0.1	tr	0	0	0	344
Molasses	tr	0	0	0	0	234
Sugar, caster	0	0	0	0	0	400
Sugar, demerara	0	0	0	0	0	394
Sugar, light muscavado	0	0	0	0	0	376
Sugar, dark muscavado	0	0	0	0	0	355
Sugar, preserving	0	0	0	0	0	400
Sugar, white	0	0	0	0	0	394
Treacle, black	0	0	0	0	0	257
Sweeteners						
Canderel	0	0	0	0	0	38
Hermesetas	0	0	0	0	0	28
Splenda	0	0	0	0	0	40

TIP: Using artificial sweeteners won't help you lose your sweet tooth, and some of them can have surprisingly laxative side effects.

SWEETS AND CHOCOLATES

Sweets and chocolates may be tempting but, by and large, do not form part of a heart-friendly diet. The one exception may be high cocoa-content chocolate (with over 70 per cent cocoa solids). Cocoa flavonoids seem to have antioxidant effects on LDLs, but the quantity of natural flavonoids in chocolate can vary a lot. It depends on the type of beans used, the way they are processed, the growing conditions … so this isn't a licence to eat loads of chocolate which is, of course, high in calories. Research continues.

TIP: Nutritional labelling which uses a percentage of the guideline daily amount (GDA) for ingredients like salt and sugar – often shown on the front of packaging in coloured boxes – can be misleading if you're not careful. Check the portions used to reach the figures (they're usually in a small font near by).

Food type	Total fat (g)	Sat (g)	Mono (g)	Poly (g)	Chol (mg)	Cal (kcal)
Aero, milk	30.8	19.7	N	N	n/k	518
After Eight mints, milk	12.1	7.6	N	N	n/k	417
Boiled sweets	tr	O	O	O	0	327
Bounty bar, milk	26.3	20.5	4.8	0.8	4	471
Caramel, Cadbury	23.3	13.9	N	N	n/k	480
Chewy sweets, e.g. Starburst	5.6	3	2.2	0.2	0	381
Coated chocolate buttons, e.g. Smarties	17.5	10.4	5.7	0.6	17e	456
Chocolate-covered caramel, average, e.g. Rolo	21.7	10.7	9.1	0.7	23	465
Chocolate, fancy and filled	21.3	11.3	8	1	11	447
Chocolate, fruit and nut	30	15	11.1	2	40	490
Chocolate, milk	30.7	18.3	9.9	1.2	23	520
Chocolate, plain	28	16.8	9	1	6	510
Chocolate, white	30.9	18.4	10	1.1	N	529
Chocolate, whole nut	37	18	15.8	1.5	50	550

TIP: Make your own delicious fruit sweets. Grind a tablespoon each of pumpkin, sunflower and sesame seeds until fine. Put them in a food processor with 350g mixed dried fruit and the grated rind of an orange. Add as much orange juice as you need to get the processor to work and blend until you have a thick ball of chopped fruit – it mustn't be runny. Spread some finely chopped hazelnuts on a plate, form the fruit paste into small balls and roll them in the hazelnuts until covered. Chill for an hour or more before serving.

Food type	Total fat (g)	Sat (g)	Mono (g)	Poly (g)	Chol (mg)	Cal (kcal)
Creme Egg	15.9	2	N	N	10	425
Flake, Cadbury	30.8	N	N	N	n/k	525
Flake, Praline, Cadbury	34.3	N	N	N	n/k	535
Fruit gums or jellies	0	0	0	0	0	324
Fruit pastilles, Rowntrees	0	0	0	0	0	350
Fudge	13.7	8.7	3.6	0.5	39	438
Kinder Bueno	37.5	N	N	N	n/k	563
Kit Kat	26	16.2	7.5	0.7	12	500
Lion bar	24.9	15.6	N	N	n/k	522
Liquorice Allsorts	5.2	3.6	1.2	0.2	0	349
Mars bar	16.7	10.3	6.7	1	8	473
Marshmallows	0	0	0	0	0	327
Milky Way	16.7	9.5	6.1	0.9	7	445
Mint Crème Chocolate, Sainsbury	25	12	9	0.8	n/k	473
Peppermints	0.7	N	N	N	0	393
Sherbet sweets	0	0	0	0	0	355
Snickers	27.8	10.9	10.9	4.3	4	497
Soft Caramel Bar, Sainsbury	22.5	13.5	7.7	1.9	n/k	453
Toffees	18.6	9.5	7.5	0.7	17	426

TIP: Make a point of keeping fresh fruit available for snacking, instead of opting for a chocolate bar. Apples, pears and bananas are all convenient to carry and contain valuable fibre. A handful of dried fruit is another good alternative.

Food type	Total fat (g)	Sat (g)	Mono (g)	Poly (g)	Chol (mg)	Cal (kcal)
Turkish delight, without nuts	0	0	0	0	0	295
Twix	24.1	11.7	11.5	0.9	4	492
Walnut Whip	25.2	13.8	N	N	n/k	495
Yorkie, milk	31.5	20.2	N	N	n/k	537
Yorkie, biscuit	26.8	16.1	N	N	n/k	510
Yorkie, biscuit and raisin	26.2	16.6	N	N	n/k	487

TIP: Make your own version of trail mix,using sultanas, raisins, chopped dried apricots and pears, and a little chopped mango; a few dried blueberries or cranberries could also be included. Keep it in an airtight jar and take it to work with you.

VEGETABLES

People who eat more vegetables have a lower incidence of cardiovascular disease. That alone is reason to ensure that you eat plenty, advice stressed by the World Health Organisation, national governments and all the organisations concerned with heart attacks and stroke. Increase the amount of vegetables you eat but be circumspect about how they are cooked – deep-fried anything will never be good news. Variety is important, and it's not enough to rely on potatoes. They don't count as one of the recommended 'five a day', in fact, largely because of their high starch content – but a bowl of crunchy salad does.

TIP: Make a coleslaw with lots of crunchy cabbage, raw onion and carrot. Don't drench all these beneficial vegetables in a high-fat dressing, though. Use zero per cent fat Greek yoghurt instead, mixed with a little low-fat mayo.

Food type	Total fat (g)	Sat (g)	Mono (g)	Poly (g)	Chol (mg)	Cal (kcal)
Asparagus, raw	0.6	0.1	0.1	0.2	0	25
Asparagus, boiled	0.8	0.1	0.2	0.3	0	26
Aubergine, raw weight	0.4	0.1	tr	0.2	0	15
Aubergine, fried in corn oil	31.9	4.1	7.9	18.5	0	302
Beansprouts, raw	0.5	0.1	0.1	0.2	0	31
Beansprouts, stir fried in blended oil	6.1	0.5	3	2.2	0	72
Beetroot, raw	0.1	tr	tr	0.1	0	36
Beetroot, boiled	0.1	tr	tr	0.1	0	46
Beetroot, pickled	0.2	tr	tr	0.1	0	28
Broad beans, frozen, boiled	0.6	0.1	0.1	0.3	0	81
Broccoli, raw weight	0.9	0.2	0.1	0.5	0	33
Broccoli, boiled	0.8	0.2	0.1	0.4	0	24
Brussels sprouts, raw	1.4	0.3	0.1	0.7	0	42
Brussels sprouts, boiled	1.3	0.3	0.1	0.7	0	35
Brussels sprouts, frozen and boiled	1.3e	0.3	0.1	0.7	0	35
Cabbage, green, raw weight	0.4	0.1	tr	0.3	0	26
Cabbage, green, boiled	0.4	0.1	tr	0.3	0	16
Cabbage, white, raw	0.2	tr	tr	0.1	0	27

Tip: Preparing vegetables carefully ensures that you retain as many nutrients as possible. Choose good-quality veg in the first place – crisp and firm – and wash, but don't soak them. Only peel them if you have to.

Food type	Total fat (g)	Sat (g)	Mono (g)	Poly (g)	Chol (mg)	Cal (kcal)
Carrots, old, raw	0.3	0.1	tr	0.2	0	35
Carrots, old, boiled	0.4	0.1	tr	0.2	0	24
Carrots, young, raw	0.5	0.1	tr	0.3	0	30
Carrots, young, boiled	0.4	0.1	tr	0.4	0	22
Carrots, canned, reheated and drained	0.3	0.1e	tr	0.2e	0	20
Cauliflower, raw	0.9	0.2	0.1	0.5	0	34
Cauliflower, boiled	0.9	0.2	0.1	0.5	0	28
Celery, raw	0.2	tr	tr	0.1	0	7
Celery, boiled	0.3	0.1	0.1	0.1	0	8
Chicory, raw	0.6	0.2	tr	0.3	0	11
Chilli peppers, raw	0.6	N	N	N	0	20
Courgette, raw weight	0.4	0.1	tr	0.2	0	18
Courgette, boiled	0.4	0.1	tr	0.2	0	19
Courgette, fried in corn oil	4.8	0.6	1.2	2.8	0	63
Cucumber, raw	0.1	tr	tr	tr	0	10
Curly kale, raw	1.6	0.2	0.1	0.9	0	33
Curly kale, boiled	1.1	0.2	0.1	0.6	0	24
Fennel, raw	0.2	tr	tr	tr	0	12
Fennel, boiled	0.2	tr	tr	tr	0	11

TIP: Don't throw away the leafy tops of celery as they add a depth of flavour to soups. Chop them and add to soups with a bean or lentil base along with the other ingredients.

Food type	Total fat (g)	Sat (g)	Mono (g)	Poly (g)	Chol (mg)	Cal (kcal)
Garlic, raw	0.6	0.1	tr	0.3	0	98
Gherkins, pickled	0.1	tr	tr	tr	0	14
Green beans / French beans, raw	0.5	0.1e	tr	0.3e	0	24
Green beans / French beans, frozen, boiled	0.1	tr	tr	tr	0	25
Karela (bitter gourd), raw weight	0.2	N	N	N	0	11
Leeks, raw	0.5	0.1	tr	0.3	0	22
Leeks, boiled	0.7	0.1	tr	0.4	0	21
Lettuce	0.5	0.1	tr	0.3	0	14
Lettuce, iceberg	0.3	tr	tr	0.2	0	13
Mange tout peas, raw	0.2	tr	tr	0.1	0	32
Mange tout peas, boiled	0.1	tr	tr	tr	0	26
Mange tout peas, stir-fried in blended oil	4.8	0.4	2.4	1.8	0	71
Marrow, raw	0.2	tr	tr	tr	0	12
Marrow, boiled	0.2	tr	tr	tr	0	9
Mixed vegetables, frozen; boiled	0.5	N	N	N	0	42
Mixed stir-fry vegetables; cooked in vegetable oil	3.6	0.3	1.8	1.3	0	64
Mushrooms, common, raw	0.5	0.1	tr	0.3	0	13
Mushrooms, fried in butter	16.2	10.7	3.9	0.5	37	157
Mushrooms, fried in corn oil	16.2	2.1	4	9.4	0	157
Mustard and cress	0.6	tr	0.2	0.2	0	13
Okra, raw	1	0.3	0.1	0.3	0	31

Food type	Total fat (g)	Sat (g)	Mono (g)	Poly (g)	Chol (mg)	Cal (kcal)
Okra, boiled	0.9	0.3	0.1	0.3	0	28
Okra, fried in corn oil	26.1	3.3	6.5	15.1	0	269
Onions, raw	0.2	tr	tr	0.1	0	36
Onions, fried in corn oil	11.2	1.4	2.8	6.5	0	164
Onions, pickled	0.2	tr	tr	0.1	0	24
Onions, pickled silverskin or cocktail	0.1	tr	tr	tr	0	15
Parsnip, raw	1.1	0.2	0.5	0.2	0	64
Parsnip, boiled	1.2	0.2	0.5	0.2	0	66
Peas, raw	1.5	0.3	0.2	0.7	0	83
Peas, boiled	1.6	0.3	0.2	0.8	0	79
Peas, frozen, boiled	0.9	0.2	0.1	0.5	0	69
Peas, canned, reheated and drained	0.9	0.2	0.1	0.4	0	80
Peas, mushy, canned	0.7	0.1	0.1	0.3	0	81
Peas, processed, canned, reheated and drained	0.7	0.1	0.1	0.3	0	99
Petits pois, frozen, boiled	0.9	0.2	0.1	0.5	0	49
Pepper, green, raw	0.3	0.1	tr	0.2	0	15
Pepper, green, boiled	0.5	0.1	tr	0.3	0	18
Pepper, red or orange, raw	0.4	0.1	tr	0.2	0	32
Pepper, red or orange, boiled	0.4	0.1	tr	0.2	0	34
Plantain, boiled	0.2	0.1	tr	0.2	0	112
Plantain, ripe, fried in vegetable oil	9.2	1	3.3	4.5	0	267

Food type	Total fat (g)	Sat (g)	Mono (g)	Poly (g)	Chol (mg)	Cal (kcal)
Potatoes						
Potatoes, new, raw weight	0.3	0.1	tr	0.1	0	70
Potatoes, new, boiled	0.3	0.1	tr	0.1	0	75
Potatoes, new, boiled in skins	0.3	0.1	tr	0.1	0	66
Potatoes, old, raw weight	0.2	tr	tr	0.1	0	75
Potatoes, old, baked, flesh and skin	0.2	tr	tr	0.1	0	136
Potatoes, old, baked, flesh only	0.1	tr	tr	0.1	0	77
Potatoes, old, mashed with butter and milk	4.3	2.8	1	0.2	12	104
Potatoes, old, roast in blended oil	4.5	0.4	2.2	1.6	0	149
Potatoes, old, roast in corn oil	4.5	0.6	1.1	2.6	0	149
Potatoes, old, roast in lard	4.5	1.8	2	0.4	4	149
Instant potato powder, made up with water	0.1	tr	tr	0.1	0	57
Instant potato powder, made up with full-cream milk	1.2	0.7	0.3	0.1	4	76
Potato croquettes, fried in blended oil	13.1	1.7	3.2	7.6	0	214

TIP: Baked potatoes make a good light meal, but do eat the skin – the fibre is valuable. Don't add butter or other high-fat toppings, either… chopped spring onions mixed with low-fat Greek yoghurt are good; so are baked beans.

Food type	Total fat (g)	Sat (g)	Mono (g)	Poly (g)	Chol (mg)	Cal (kcal)
Potato fritters, battered, oven baked	8.5	3.8	3.3	1	1	185
Potato waffles, frozen, cooked	8.2	1	2	4.7	0	200
Chips						
Chips, home-made, fried in blended oil	6.7	0.6	3.3	2.4	0	189
Chips, home-made, fried in corn oil	6.7	0.9	1.7	3.9	0	189
Chips, home-made, fried in dripping	6.7	3.7	2.5	0.2	6	189
Chips, shop, fried in blended oil	12.4	1.1	6.2	4.5	0	239
Chips, shop, fried in vegetable oil	12.4	3.6	5.3	3.1	0	239
Chips, shop, fried in dripping	12.4	6.8	4.6	0.3	11	239
French fries, from fast-food shops	15.5	5.8	6.9	2.1	N	280
French fries, straight cut, frozen, fried in blended oil	13.5	1.2	6.7	4.9	0	273
French fries, straight cut, frozen, fried in corn oil	13.5	2.5	3.4	7	0	273
French fries, straight cut, frozen, fried in dripping	13.5	7.5	5	0.3	12	273
French fries, fine cut, frozen, fried in blended oil	21.3	1.8	10.6	7.8	0	364
French fries, fine cut, frozen, fried in corn oil	21.3	4	5.4	11	0	364

Food type	Total fat (g)	Sat (g)	Mono (g)	Poly (g)	Chol (mg)	Cal (kcal)
French fries, fine cut, frozen, fried in dripping	21.3	11.8	7.9	0.5	0	364
Microwave chips, cooked	9.6	N	N	N	0	221
Oven chips, frozen, baked	4.2	1.8	1.6	0.6	0	162
Pumpkin, raw, flesh only	0.2	0.1	tr	tr	0	13
Pumpkin, flesh only, boiled	0.3	0.1	tr	tr	0	13
Quorn, pieces	3.2	0.6	0.7	1.9	0	92
Radish, red, raw	0.2	0.1	tr	0.1	0	12
Runner beans, raw	0.4	0.1	tr	0.2	0	22
Runner beans, boiled	0.5	0.1	tr	0.3	0	18
Shallots, raw	0.2	tr	tr	0.1	0	20
Spinach, raw	0.8	0.1	0.1	0.5	0	25
Spinach, boiled	0.8	0.1	0.1	0.5	0	19
Spinach, frozen and boiled	0.8e	0.1	0.1	0.5	0	21
Spring greens, raw	1	0.1	0.1	0.6	0	33
Spring greens, boiled	0.7	0.1	0.1	0.4	0	20
Spring onions, raw	0.5	0.1	0.1	0.2	0	23
Swede, raw weight, flesh only	0.3	tr	tr	0.2	0	24
Swede, boiled	0.3	tr	tr	0.1	0	11
Sweet potato, raw weight	0.3	0.1	tr	0.1	0	87

TIP: Grate some raw carrots, add some grated apple and toss the mixture in a little oil and lemon dressing – a fresh salad and a good accompaniment for grilled meat.

Food type	Total fat (g)	Sat (g)	Mono (g)	Poly (g)	Chol (mg)	Cal (kcal)
Sweet potato, boiled	0.3	0.1	tr	0.1	0	84
Sweetcorn, baby, canned, drained	0.4	N	N	N	0	23
Sweetcorn, canned kernels, drained	1.2	0.2	0.3	0.5	0	122
Sweetcorn, boiled on the cob	2.3	0.2	0.3	0.5	0	111
Tomatoes, raw	0.3	0.1	0.1	0.2	0	17
Tomatoes, canned	0.1	tr	tr	tr	0	16
Tomatoes, fried in corn oil	7.7	1	1.9	4.5	0	91
Tomatoes, grilled	0.3	1.1	0.1	0.2	0	20
Turnip, raw weight, flesh only	0.3	tr	tr	0.2	0	23
Turnip, boiled	0.2	tr	tr	0.1	0	12
Watercress	1	0.3	0.1	0.4	0	22
Yam, raw weight	0.3	0.1	tr	0.1	0	114
Yam, boiled	0.3	0.1	tr	0.1	0	133
Vegetable dishes						
Bubble and squeak, fried in vegetable oil	9.1	1.1	4.7	2.9	0	125
Cauliflower cheese, made with semi-skimmed milk	6.5	2.9	1.7	1.4	11	102
Garlic mushrooms (uncoated)	14.4	8.9	3.5	0.8	36	140
Pancakes stuffed with vegetables	7.6	2.2	2.3	2.6	27	137
Ratatouille, frozen, cooked	6.6	0.8	1.6	3.6	0	78

Food type	Total fat (g)	Sat (g)	Mono (g)	Poly (g)	Chol (mg)	Cal (kcal)
Sauerkraut	tr	tr	tr	tr	0	9
Tsatsiki (cucumber and yoghurt)	4.9	2.8	1.4	0.3	N	66
Salads						
Coleslaw, with mayo	26.4	3.9	6	15.3	26	258
Coleslaw, reduced calorie	4.5	0.5	1.5	2.2	0	67
Green salad	0.3	0.1	tr	0.1	0	12
Potato salad, with mayo	26.5	3.9	6.1	15.4	26	287
Rice salad	7.5	1.1	3.8	2.1	0	165
For dried beans etc., see *Beans, pulses and grains*						

TIP: Skinning peppers, particularly green ones, can make them more digestible. Cut the peppers in half and remove the seeds. Rub them with a little olive oil (use kitchen paper to do this) and place them skin side uppermost in a roasting dish. Cook them in a medium oven until the skins begin to blister and blacken. Remove them from the oven and allow to cool until you can handle them. Peel them carefully, using a knife to tease the skin away from the flesh. A mixture of coloured peppers, skinned like this and then sliced, makes a delicious salad and needs no dressing.

VEGETARIAN

Theoretically vegetarians should be at lower risk of cardiovascular disease, but this has yet to be clearly demonstrated. Though many vegetarians do have lower LDL levels, they have lower levels of HDL too. There is some evidence that people who are vegetarian or vegan have higher levels of homocysteine, the inflammatory protein which is removed from the body by various substances including vitamin B12. This is naturally found in animal products, so using B12 supplements – or selecting food fortified with it – may be worthwhile. Marmite, for instance, contains B12. It is also worth considering the high saturated fat content of items such as vegetarian cheese and opting for lower-fat tofu whenever possible.

TIP: If you're vegetarian, you will probably find it easier to incorporate more soya into your diet, as many vegetarians often use soya products; if you don't, give them a try.

Food type	Total fat (g)	Sat (g)	Mono (g)	Poly (g)	Chol (mg)	Cal (kcal)
Beanburger, soya, fried in vegetable oil	11	1.5	4.2	4	33	193
Cannelloni, Tuscan Four Bean, Cauldron Foods	4.5	2.5	N	N	N	116
Cheddar, vegetarian	32	20.8	8.7	1.2	105	390
Falafel	9.8	1.6	N	N	N	203
Ghee, vegetable	99.4	48.4	37	9.7	0	895
Mushroom burgers, Cauldron Foods	6.3	0.8	N	N	N	143
Nut roast	23.5	3.6	12.8	5.8	0	333
Pâté, Chickpea & Black Olive, Cauldron Foods	10.5	1.3	N	N	N	171
Pâté, Roasted Parsnip & Carrot, Cauldron Foods	6.7	2.9	N	N	N	115
Quorn burgers with cheese	7	3	N	N	N	163
Quorn, pieces	3.2	0.6	0.7	1.9	0	92
Sausages, Glamorgan, Cauldron Foods	9.2	3.4	N	N	N	162
Sausages, Mushroom & Herb, Cauldron Foods	6.8	4.1	N	N	N	134
Shepherd's pie, vegetable	4.9	2	1.2	1.4	7	101

TIP: Good vegetable sources of omega-3 fatty acids are walnuts, rapeseed oil and linseeds (also called flaxseeds), soya beans and dark green vegetables.

Food type	Total fat (g)	Sat (g)	Mono (g)	Poly (g)	Chol (mg)	Cal (kcal)
Soya milk, sweetened, plus calcium	2.4	0.4	0.5	1.4	0	43
Soya milk, unsweetened	1.6	0.2	0.3	1.1	0	26
Soya milk, unsweetened, Alpro light	1.2	0.2	0.3	0.7	0	21
Soya yoghurt, fruit	1.8	0.3	0.4	1.1	0	73
Spinach & Sweetcorn Crisp Bakes, Cauldron Foods	11.8	3.5	N	N	N	222
Suet, vegetable	87.9	45	26.3	12.8	0	836
Sweet Potato & Aubergine Balti, Cauldron Foods	1.5	0.1	N	N	N	100
Tofu, marinated, Cauldron Foods	18.3	2.6	N	N	N	241
Tofu, steamed	4.2	0.5	0.8	2	0	73
Tofu, steamed and fried	17.7	N	N	N	0	261
Vegeburger, grilled	11.1	N	N	N	N	196
Vegetable and cheese crispbakes (coated)	14	4.6	4.4	3	N	240
Vegetable bake, with cheese sauce	7.2	2.9	2.1	1.7	11	131
Vegetable casserole (no pulses)	0.4	0.1	0.1	0.2	0	52

TIP: You may be taking in more saturated fat than you think if you're vegetarian, so check your intake of dairy products. It's easy to eat a lot of cheese, especially when you use it in cooking.

Food type	Total fat (g)	Sat (g)	Mono (g)	Poly (g)	Chol (mg)	Cal (kcal)
Vegetable chilli	0.6	0.1	0.1	0.2	tr	56
Vegetable curry	3	N	N	N	tr	102
Vegetable Kiev	13.7	5	5.2	2.8	13	229
Vegetable quiche	14.5	5.4	6.4	3.2	15	226
Vegetable pasty	16.5	2.2	2.3	2.6	27	289
Vegetable pie	8.4	2.6	3.1	2.2	4	159
Vegetarian pizza	6.9	N	N	N	N	216
Vegetarian sausages	9.4	2.3	4.1	1.9	0	179
For dried beans etc., see *Beans, pulses and grains*						

TIP: Strict vegetarians and vegans, who don't eat dairy products, may need to take calcium supplements, as calcium is vital for your health. Always use soya milk reinforced with calcium.

FAST FOOD AND TAKEAWAYS

If you only eat takeaways or fast food very infrequently and make sensible choices, you probably don't need to worry too much. However, if you use fast food or takeaway restaurants regularly, even if it's just to pick up a cappuccino on the way to work, think seriously about reducing the number of your visits and amending the choices you make. Menus and portion sizes vary, but use the figures in this section as a guide. Remember, too, that calorie counts can be high. You can easily eat half your daily recommended calorie intake in one quick visit to a coffee shop if you're not careful.

TIP: It's been reported that more than 2 billion takeaways are bought in the UK each year. One of the best ways to improve your diet instantly is to cut back on these.

Food type	Total fat (g)	Sat (g)	Mono (g)	Poly (g)	Chol (mg)	Cal (kcal)
Fish and chips, etc.						
Chips, fried in blended oil	12.4	1.1	6.2	4.5	0	239
Chips, fried in vegetable oil	12.4	3.6	5.3	3.1	0	239
Chips, fried in dripping	12.4	6.8	4.6	0.3	11	239
French fries	15.5	5.8	6.9	2.1	N	280
Eel, jellied	7.1	1.9	3.5	1	79	98
Cod in batter, fried in blended oil	15.4	1.6	5.5	7.5	N	247
Cod roe, hard, coated and fried in blended oil	11.9	1.6	4.1	5.7	315	202
Rock salmon (dogfish), in batter, fried in blended oil	21.9	2.9	8	9.9	N	295
Scampi in breadcrumbs, fried in blended oil	13.6	1.4	5.1	6.4	110	237
Mushy peas	0.7	0.1	0.1	0.3	0	81
Saveloy, without batter	22.3	7.5	9.8	3.6	78	296
Fried white bread, cooked in lard	32.2	12.5	13.4	2.9	tr	498
Indian food						
Chicken curry, average	9.8	2.9	4	2.5	37	145
Chicken tikka masala	10.6	3.6	4.3	2.3	46	157
Chickpea dhal	6.1	0.7	2.6	2.2	0	154
Fish curry, Bangladeshi	8	N	N	N	N	127
Meat samosas	17.3	4.5	7	4.8	20	272
Pakora and bahjia, vegetable	14.7	1	7.6	4.8	0	235
Prawn curry, average	8.5	1.4	3.8	2.9	144	117

Food type	Total fat (g)	Sat (g)	Mono (g)	Poly (g)	Chol (mg)	Cal (kcal)
Vegetable samosa	9.3	N	N	N	0	217
Pilau rice, plain	4.6	2.6	1.1	0.5	10	142
Chapati, made with fat	12.8	N	N	N	N	328
Chapati, made without fat	1	0.1	0.1	0.4	0	202
Poppadoms	38.8	8	16.5	12.5	2	501
Lassi, yoghurt drink, sweetened	0.9	0.6	0.2	tr	N	62
Chinese food						
Beef chow mein	6	1.3	3.1	1.4	N	136
Chicken chow mein	7.2	1.2	3.9	1.8	13	147
Chicken satay	10.3	3	4.3	2.5	57	191
Crispy duck, Chinese style	24.2	7.2	12.3	3.4	63	331
Fish balls, Chinese, steamed	0.5	N	N	N	N	74
Prawns with vegetables, Szechuan	4.7	0.7	2.4	1.4	56	83
Spring rolls, with meat	16.4	3.8	7.1	4.8	7	242
Stir-fried vegetables	4.1	0.8	2.2	0.6	1	52
Sweet and sour chicken	10	1.3	5.2	3	24	194
Sweet and sour pork	8.6	2	3.9	2	51	177
Sweet and sour sauce, takeaway	3.4	N	N	N	0	157
Egg-fried rice	4.9	0.6	2.3	1.3	19	186
Prawn crackers	39	3.6	22.4	11	0	570
Middle-Eastern and Greek						
Doner kebabs, meat only	31.4	15.3	12	1.4	94	377
Doner kebabs, with pitta and salad	16.2	7.8	6.1	0.9	47	255

Food type	Total fat (g)	Sat (g)	Mono (g)	Poly (g)	Chol (mg)	Cal (kcal)
Hummus, average	19	2	9.6	6.5	0	202
Moussaka	8.3	2.9	3.6	1.1	26	140
Shish kebab, meat only	10	3.9	4.3	0.8	90	206
Shish kebab, with pitta and salad	4.1	1.5	1.6	0.5	33	155
Taramasalata, average	52.9	4.1	29.3	16.7	25	504
Tsatsiki, average	4.9	2.8	1.4	0.3	N	66
Greek pastries, average, including baklava	17	N	N	N	N	322
Pizzas						
Cheese and tomato pizza, deep pan	7.5	3.1	2.4	1.3	13	249
Cheese and tomato pizza, thin base	10.3	4.8	3.1	1.3	22	277
Pizza with fish-based topping, average	7.5	3.2	2.5	1.3	25	226
Ham and pineapple pizza	8.6	N	N	N	N	260
Pizza with meat-based topping, average	10.3	4	3.7	1.5	19	255
Vegetarian pizza	6.9	N	N	N	N	216

TIP: Fast foods are often a source of both saturated and trans fats. For this reason alone it's wise to limit – or stop – your consumption of them. Trans fats are thought to be even worse than saturated fats for increasing the body's levels of 'bad cholesterol'.

Food type	Total fat (g)	Sat (g)	Mono (g)	Poly (g)	Chol (mg)	Cal (kcal)
Fast food restaurants						
Milkshake, thick, takeaway, average	1.8	1.2	0.4	0.1	11	88
Big Mac (including bun, etc.)	10.7	4.6	4.4	1.6	23	228
Cheesburger (including bun, etc.)	11.8	6.2	5.4	0.9	32	259
Chicken burger (including bun, etc.)	10.8	N	N	N	N	267
Hamburger (including bun, etc.)	9.6	4	4.2	0.8	40	243
Quarterpounder with cheese (including bun, etc.)	13	6.4	5.6	0.9	33	250
Whopper burger (including bun, etc.)	14.8	4.4	5.4	4.2	31	241
Chicken nuggets	13	3.3	6.8	2.2	55	265
Hamburger buns	5	1.1	1.3	1.1	0	264
Sandwiches						
Bacon, lettuce and tomato, white bread, average	12.4	2.8	3.8	4.9	18	235
Cheddar cheese and pickle, white bread, average	14.9	7.4	4.1	2.3	30	290
Chicken salad, white bread, average	5.3	1.2	1.8	1.9	26	175
Egg mayo, white bread, average	12	2.4	3.7	4.9	111	248
Ham salad, white bread, average	4.5	0.9	1.4	1.8	12	167
Tuna mayo, white bread, average	10.5	1.7	2.7	5.4	23	237

Food type	Total fat (g)	Sat (g)	Mono (g)	Poly (g)	Chol (mg)	Cal (kcal)
Chicken and bacon, deep fill, Asda	9.3	2.2	N	N	n/k	239
Chicken salad, Marks & Spencer	4.1	1.0	n/k	n/k	n/k	155
Chicken & sweetcorn, Marks & Spencer	6.8	0.9	n/k	n/k	n/k	185
Ploughman's, Marks & Spencer	16.1	8.7	n/k	n/k	n/k	250
Prawn mayo, Asda	14.5	1.7	N	N	n/k	253
Tuna and cucumber, 'good for you', Asda	1.6	0.4	0.8	0.4	n/k	144
Tuna and sweetcorn, Asda	13.5	1.6	N	N	n/k	246
Chicken salad wrap, Sainsbury	12.4	3.2	N	N	n/k	233
Falafel and hummus wrap, Sainsbury	8	2.2	N	N	n/k	196
Peking Duck wrap, Asda	7.6	2.4	3.4	1.4	n/k	219
Tuna Crunch wrap, Sainsbury	3.7	1.8	N	N	n/k	140
Coffee shop drinks – Starbucks (by portion size)						
Cappuccino, tall, whole milk	6.4	4	n/k	n/k	26	122
Cappuccino, tall, skimmed milk	0	0	n/k	n/k	4	76

TIP: Some apparently 'healthy' options can be deceptively high in both fat and calories. Watch the type of salad dressing you choose.

Food type	Total fat (g)	Sat (g)	Mono (g)	Poly (g)	Chol (mg)	Cal (kcal)
Cappuccino, grande, whole milk	7.7	4.8	n/k	n/k	31	153
Cappuccino, grande, skimmed milk	0	0	n/k	n/k	5	96
Cappuccino, venti, whole milk	10.7	6.7	n/k	n/k	43	207
Cappuccino, venti, skimmed milk	0	0	n/k	n/k	7	129
Caffe Latte, tall, whole milk	10.6	6.6	n/k	n/k	43	200
Caffe Latte, tall, skimmed milk	0	0	n/k	n/k	6	122
Caffe Latte, grande, whole milk	13.8	8.6	n/k	n/k	56	265
Caffe Latte, grande, skimmed milk	0	0	n/k	n/k	8	163
Caffe Latte, venti, whole milk	17.9	11.2	n/k	n/k	73	341
Caffe Latte, venti, skimmed milk	0	0	n/k	n/k	11	208
Caffe Mocha with whip, tall, whole milk	17.3	10	n/k	n/k	57	313
Caffe Mocha with whip, tall, skimmed milk	9.3	5.4	n/k	n/k	35	255

TIP: Sandwiches are a great substitute for fast food snacking at lunchtime, but make your own. You control the ingredients, and can avoid high-fat fillings and dressings. Don't forget that fillings such as tomatoes that make the bread soggy don't travel well. You can always take moist fillings separately and assemble your sandwich at lunchtime.

Food type	Total fat (g)	Sat (g)	Mono (g)	Poly (g)	Chol (mg)	Cal (kcal)
Caffe Mocha with whip, grande, whole milk	21.4	12.3	n/k	n/k	69	396
Caffe Mocha with whip, grande, skimmed milk	11.6	6.7	n/k	n/k	43	324
Caffe Mocha with whip, venti, whole milk	25.3	14.3	n/k	n/k	80	484
Caffe Mocha with whip, venti, skimmed milk	12.2	6.8	n/k	n/k	44	388
Caramel Macchiato, tall, whole milk	10.4	6	n/k	n/k	32	244
Caramel Macchiato, tall, skimmed milk	0.8	0.5	n/k	n/k	6	173
Caramel Macchiato, grande, whole milk	13.6	8.5	n/k	n/k	53	319
Caramel Macchiato, grande, skimmed milk	2.1	1.3	n/k	n/k	13	234
Caramel Macchiato, venti, whole milk	17.4	10.9	n/k	n/k	69	390
Caramel Macchiato, venti, skimmed milk	2.1	1.3	n/k	n/k	15	277
Hot chocolate with whip, tall, whole milk	18.7	10.7	n/k	n/k	60	357
Hot chocolate with whip, tall, skimmed milk	9.5	5.4	n/k	n/k	35	289

Food type	Total fat (g)	Sat (g)	Mono (g)	Poly (g)	Chol (mg)	Cal (kcal)
Hot chocolate with whip, grande, whole milk	23.5	13.4	n/k	n/k	75	448
Hot chocolate with whip, grande, skimmed milk	11.8	6.7	n/k	n/k	44	362
Hot chocolate with whip, venti, whole milk	27	15.2	n/k	n/k	85	549
Hot chocolate with whip, venti, skimmed milk	12.3	6.8	n/k	n/k	45	441
Coffee Frappuccino with whip and syrup, tall	11.3	7.4	n/k	n/k	47	313
Coffee Frappuccino with whip and syrup, grande	15.8	10.3	n/k	n/k	65	422
Coffee Frappuccino with whip and syrup, venti	16.3	10.7	n/k	n/k	68	484
Mocha Frappuccino with whip and syrup, tall	11.9	7.5	n/k	n/k	47	331
Mocha Frappuccino with whip and syrup, grande	16.3	10.4	n/k	n/k	65	440
Mocha Frappuccino with whip and syrup, venti	17.6	10.9	n/k	n/k	68	534

FURTHER READING

Before the Heart Attacks, Dr Robert H. Superko with Laura Tucker, Rodale, 2004

Colllins Need to Know GI/GL, 2006

Collins Need to Know Calorie Counting, 2007

Collins Gem Calorie Counter, revised edition 2006

Collins Gem GI, 2005

Eat, Drink and Be Healthy, Walter Willett, M.D., The Free Press, 2005

The Food Bible, Judith Wills, Quadrille, 2001

Healthy Eating for Lower Cholesterol, Daniel Green and Catherine Collins, Kyle Cathie, 2007

Healthy Eating for Your Heart, Paul Gayler and Jacqui Lynas, Kyle Cathie, 2003

Low-Cholesterol Cooking for Health, edited by Christine France, Southwater, 2003

Nutrition for Life, Lisa Hark and Darwin Deen, Dorling Kindersley, 2005

Real Fast Food, Nigel Slater, Penguin, 2006 (for those who claim they don't have time to cook!)

Understanding Cholesterol, Mike Laker, Family Doctor Books, 2006 edition

USEFUL ADDRESSES

The Blood Pressure Association
60 Cranmer Terrace
London SW17 0QS
020 8772 4994
www.bpassoc.org.uk

The British Dietetic Association
5th Floor, Charles House
148/9 Great Charles Street
Queensway
Birmingham B3 3HT
0121 200 8080
www.bda.uk.com

British Heart Foundation
14 Fitzhardinge Street
London W1H 6DG
020 7935 0185
www.bhf.org.uk

British Nutrition Foundation
High Holborn House
52-54 High Holborn
London WC1V 6RQ
020 7404 6504
www.nutrition.org.uk

Chest, Heart and Stroke Scotland
65 North Castle Street
Edinburgh EH2 3LT
0131 225 6963
www.chss.org.uk

Diabetes UK
10 Parkway
London NW1 7AA
Careline 0845 1202960
020 7424 1000
www.diabetes.org.uk

H·E·A·R·T UK
7 North Road
Maidenhead
Berkshire, SL6 1PE
01628 628638
www.heartuk.org.uk
(familial hypercholesterolaemia)

Northern Ireland Chest, Heart and Stroke Association
22 Great Victoria Street,
Belfast BT2 7LX
028 9032 0184
0845 3033100
www.nichsa.com

Quit
211 Old Street
London EC1V 9NR
020 7251 1551
www.quit.org.uk
(stopping smoking)

The Stroke Association
Stroke House
240 City Road
London EC1V 2PR
020 7566 0300
www.stroke.org.uk

USEFUL WEBSITES

- www.nhsdirect.nhs.uk
- www.bhsoc.org – British Hypertension Society, professional site aimed at doctors but with some useful info
- www.healthnet.org.uk (the Coronary Prevention Group)
- www.eatwell.gov.uk
- www.weightlossresources.co.uk
- www.bbc.co.uk/health
- www.bupa.co.uk – for good general health info, basic and easy to understand. Sensible.
- www.netdoctor.co.uk/health_advice
- www.5aday.nhs.uk – about fruit and veg
- www.vegsoc.org – for vegetarians
- www.salt.gov.uk – advice about your salt intake
- www.omega3-info.com